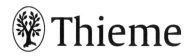

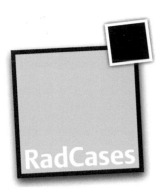

RadCases Gastrointestinal Imaging
Second Edition

Edited by

Stephen Thomas, MD
Associate Professor of Radiology
Section of Abdominal Imaging
The University of Chicago
Chicago, Illinois

Jonathan M. Lorenz, MD, FSIR
Professor of Radiology
Section of Interventional Radiology
The University of Chicago
Chicago, Illinois

Series Editors

Jonathan M. Lorenz, MD, FSIR
Professor of Radiology
Section of Interventional Radiology
The University of Chicago
Chicago, Illinois

Hector Ferral, MD
Senior Medical Educator
NorthShore University HealthSystem
Evanston, Illinois

552 illustrations

Thieme
New York • Stuttgart • Delhi • Rio de Janeiro

Library of Congress Cataloging-in-Publication Data
Names: Thomas, Stephen, 1971- editor. | Lorenz, Jonathan, editor.
Title: RadCases gastrointestinal imaging / [edited] by Stephen Thomas, Jonathan M. Lorenz.
Other titles: Gastrointestinal imaging (Lorenz) | RadCases.
Description: Second edition. | New York : Thieme, 2020. | Series: RadCases | Preceded by Gastrointestinal imaging / edited by Jonathan Lorenz. c2011. | Includes bibliographical references and index. | Summary: "RadCases Gastrointestinal Imaging Second Edition by Stephen Thomas and Jonathan M. Lorenz expands on the rich study experience that has been tried, tested, and popularized by radiology residents around the world. This new edition includes important variations on prior cases, updated diagnostic and management strategies, and new pathological entities. One hundred new, carefully selected GI cases are focused on helping radiology residents navigate and assimilate a daunting volume of digestive-related information. For maximum ease of self-assessment, each case begins with the clinical presentation on the right-hand page; study that and then turn the page for imaging findings, differential diagnoses with the definitive diagnosis, essential facts, pearls and pitfalls, and more" – Provided by publisher.
Identifiers: LCCN 2020001839 (print) | LCCN 2020001840 (ebook) | ISBN 9781626238688 (paperback) | ISBN 9781626238695 (ebook)
Subjects: MESH: Gastrointestinal Diseases–diagnostic imaging | Radiography | Diagnosis, Differential | Gastrointestinal Tract–diagnostic imaging | Case Reports
Classification: LCC RC804.D52 (print) | LCC RC804.D52 (ebook) | NLM WI 141 | DDC 616.3/3075–dc23
LC record available at https://lccn.loc.gov/2020001839
LC ebook record available at https://lccn.loc.gov/2020001840

Important note: Medicine is an ever-changing science undergoing continual development. Research and clinical experience are continually expanding our knowledge, in particular our knowledge of proper treatment and drug therapy. Insofar as this book mentions any dosage or application, readers may rest assured that the authors, editors, and publishers have made every effort to ensure that such references are in accordance with **the state of knowledge at the time of production of the book.**

Nevertheless, this does not involve, imply, or express any guarantee or responsibility on the part of the publishers in respect to any dosage instructions and forms of applications stated in the book. **Every user is requested to examine carefully** the manufacturers' leaflets accompanying each drug and to check, if necessary in consultation with a physician or specialist, whether the dosage schedules mentioned therein or the contraindications stated by the manufacturers differ from the statements made in the present book. Such examination is particularly important with drugs that are either rarely used or have been newly released on the market. Every dosage schedule or every form of application used is entirely at the user's own risk and responsibility. The authors and publishers request every user to report to the publishers any discrepancies or inaccuracies noticed. If errors in this work are found after publication, errata will be posted at www.thieme.com on the product description page.

Some of the product names, patents, and registered designs referred to in this book are in fact registered trademarks or proprietary names even though specific reference to this fact is not always made in the text. Therefore, the appearance of a name without designation as proprietary is not to be construed as a representation by the publisher that it is in the public domain.

Copyright © 2020 by Thieme Medical Publishers, Inc.
Thieme Publishers New York
333 Seventh Avenue, New York, NY 10001 USA
+1 800 782 3488, customerservice@thieme.com

Thieme Publishers Stuttgart
Rüdigerstrasse 14, 70469 Stuttgart, Germany
+49 [0]711 8931 421, customerservice@thieme.de

Thieme Publishers Delhi
A-12, Second Floor, Sector-2, Noida-201301
Uttar Pradesh, India
+91 120 45 566 00, customerservice@thieme.in

Thieme Revinter Publicações Ltda.
Rua do Matoso, 170 – Tijuca
Rio de Janeiro RJ 20270-135 – Brasil
+55 21 2563-9702
www.thiemerevinter.com.br

Cover design: Thieme Publishing Group
Typesetting by Absolute Service, Inc.
Printed in the United States by King Printing Co., Inc.
5 4 3 2 1

ISBN 978-1-62623-868-8

Also available as an e-book:
eISBN 978-1-62623-869-5

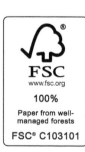

FSC
www.fsc.org
100%
Paper from well-managed forests
FSC® C103101

Dedicated to my sons Andrew and Oliver: thank you for your love, smiles, and giggles. Your endless curiosity and eagerness to learn helped me become a better teacher and researcher. You taught me just the mere act of reading a book does not make one a teacher. It's about enthusiasm, acting, repetition, abstraction, and creating. I hope I am able to impart in you the love for teaching your grandma Rosaline gave me. Perhaps, one day you will understand that teaching is what ultimately makes one an expert. Brighten your curiosity, learn and understand, don't let mistakes stop you, create the new, better what you do, and teach what you have learned. Love, Dad

– ST

Dedicated to my wife, Cynthia, for your love and support, and to my kids, Anna and Matthew: your dreams, hard work, and successes inspire me.

– JML

Series Preface

As enthusiastic partners in radiology education, we continue our mission to ease the exhaustion and frustration shared by residents and the families of residents engaged in radiology training! In launching the second edition of the RadCases series, our intent is to expand rather than replace this already rich study experience that has been tried, tested, and popularized by residents around the world. In each subspecialty edition, we serve up 100 new, carefully chosen cases to raise the bar in our effort to assist residents in tackling the daunting task of assimilating massive amounts of information. RadCases second edition primes and expands on concepts found in the first edition with important variations on prior cases, updated diagnostic and management strategies, and new pathological entities. Our continuing goal is to combine the popularity and portability of printed books with the adaptability, exceptional quality, and interactive features of an electronic case-based format. The new cases will be added to the existing electronic database to enrich the interactive environment of high-quality images that allows residents to arrange study sessions, quickly extract and master information, and prepare for theme-based radiology conferences.

We owe a debt of gratitude to our own residents and to the many radiology trainees who have helped us create, adapt, and improve the format and content of RadCases by weighing in with suggestions for new cases, functions, and formatting. Back by popular demand is the concise, point-by-point presentation of the Essential Facts of each case in an easy-to-read, bulleted format, and a short, critical differential starting with the actual diagnosis. This approach is easy on exhausted eyes and encourages repeated priming of important information during quick reviews, a process we believe is critical to radiology education. New since the prior edition is the addition of a question-and-answer section for each case to reinforce key concepts.

The intent of the printed books is to encourage repeated priming in the use of critical information by providing a portable group of exceptional core cases to master. Unlike the authors of other case-based radiology review books, we removed the guesswork by providing clear annotations and descriptions for all images. In our opinion, there is nothing worse than being unable to locate a subtle finding on a poorly reproduced image even after one knows the final diagnosis.

The electronic cases expand on the printed book and provide a comprehensive review of the entire specialty. Thousands of cases are strategically designed to increase the resident's knowledge by providing exposure to a spectrum of case examples—from basic to advanced—and by exploring "Aunt Minnies," unusual diagnoses, and variability within a single diagnosis. The search engine allows the resident to create individualized, daily study lists that are not limited by factors such as radiology subsection. For example, tailor today's study list to cases involving tuberculosis and include cases in every subspecialty and every system of the body. Or study only thoracic cases, including those with links to cardiology, nuclear medicine, and pediatrics. Or study only musculoskeletal cases. The choice is yours.

As enthusiastic partners in this project, we started small and, with the encouragement, talent, and guidance of Timothy Hiscock and William Lamsback at Thieme Medical Publishers, we have further raised the bar in our effort to assist residents in tackling the daunting task of assimilating massive amounts of information. We are passionate about continuing this journey and will continue to expand the series, adapt cases based on direct feedback from residents, and increase the features intended for board review and self-assessment. First and foremost, we thank our medical students, residents, and fellows for allowing us the privilege to participate in their educational journey.

Jonathan M. Lorenz, MD, FSIR
Hector Ferral, MD

Preface

The gastrointestinal (GI) component of Thieme's RadCases series covers the spectrum of common and uncommon GI diagnosis an abdominal imager would encounter in their day-to-day practice. For this second edition, cases have been chosen from our imaging archive that had classic imaging findings, posed an imaging dilemma, or were misdiagnosed. A total of 100 cases are presented with annotated images from computed tomography, magnetic resonance imaging, fluoroscopic studies, positron emission tomography, and ultrasound. The multimodality approach allows the reader to understand how the same entity has different imaging features on various modalities, help choose the appropriate imaging modality, and provide a concise differential diagnosis utilizing different studies.

Cases are presented as unknowns with differential diagnosis and essential facts. Multiple choice questions help prepare the test taker and reinforce concepts for the clinical radiologist. The Pearls and Pitfalls section highlights common case mimics that may lead to a misdiagnosis.

Case 1

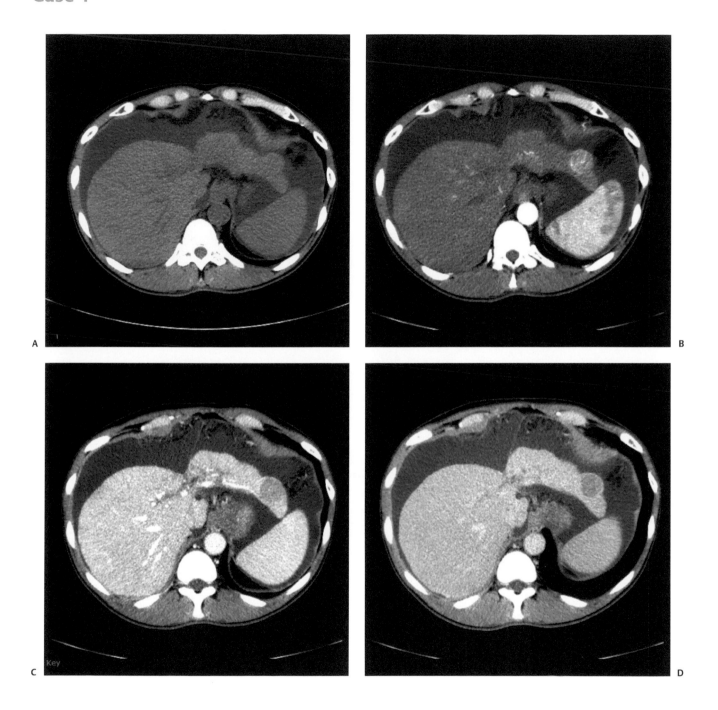

A   B

C   D

■ Clinical Presentation

A 58-year-old man with hepatitis C virus–related cirrhosis and elevated alfa-fetoprotein.

■ Imaging Findings

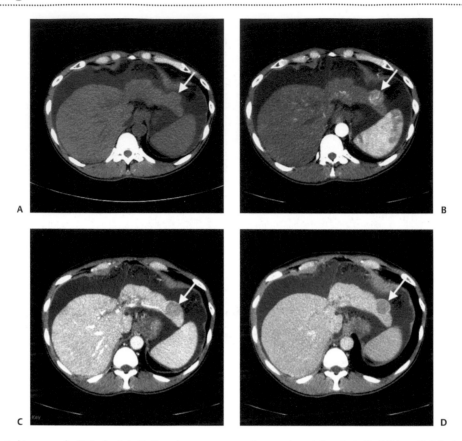

(A) Unenhanced computed tomography (CT) of a cirrhotic liver shows a mass causing a contour deformity in the left hepatic lobe (*arrow*). Note the nodular liver contour and ascites from liver failure. **(B)** Arterial phase CT shows brisk enhancement of the partially exophytic mass (*arrow*). **(C)** Portal venous phase CT shows washout of the mass (*arrow*). **(D)** Delayed phase CT shows subtle capsule around the mass (*arrow*).

■ Differential Diagnosis

- ***Hepatocellular carcinoma (HCC):*** A primary cancer of the liver that occurs in the setting of chronic liver disease. The enhancement pattern in the setting cirrhosis and liver failure is diagnostic of HCC.
- *Hepatic adenoma:* A benign lesion that can be hypervascular on arterial phase and show varying degrees of washout. It can contain varying amounts tumoral fat. It tends to occur in females and is associated with contraceptive use.
- *Hypervascular metastasis:* Renal cell carcinoma, thyroid carcinoma, neuroendocrine carcinoma, and some adenocarcinomas can be hypervascular and show washout. They can mimic a primary hepatic neoplasm.

■ Essential Facts

- CT is used to screen for HCC in the setting of chronic liver disease.
- Lesions with arterial enhancement and portal venous or delayed washout are diagnostic of HCC in the setting of chronic liver disease.
- LiRads is a classification system for liver lesions.

■ Other Imaging Findings

- Magnetic resonance imaging can be excellent in screening for HCC. It can detect intralesional fat, lesions may be T2 hyperintense, and show similar contrast enhancement characteristics as CT.
- Ultrasound is used frequently as a screening tool. Lesions can be hyperechoic, isoechoic, or hypoechoic to hepatic parenchyma. Detecting HCC in a very nodular liver is difficult and operator dependent.

✓ Pearls and ✗ Pitfalls

- ✓ Hepatic lesion with arterial enhancement and portal-venous or delayed washout in the setting of cirrhosis is characteristic of HCC.
- ✓ On a per-patient basis, the sensitivity of CT to detect HCC is 74–100%.
- ✓ Well-differentiated HCC can contain fat.
- ✗ Identification of HCC requires an arterial phase CT and a delayed phase CT as HCC can be iso-attenuating to liver on portal venous phase alone.
- ✗ Atypical HCC may not have avid arterial enhancement but can have washout.

Case 2

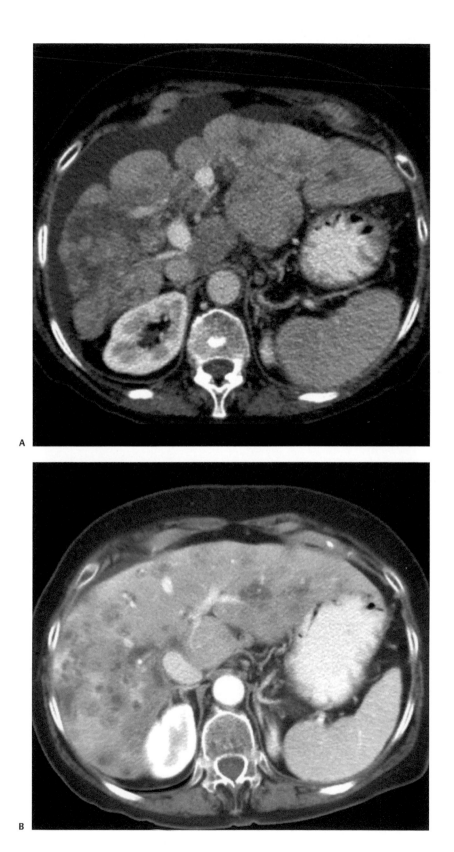

A

B

■ **Clinical Presentation**

A 48-year-old female with history of breast cancer presents with elevated liver enzymes.

■ **Imaging Findings**

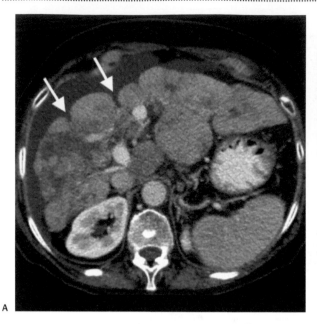 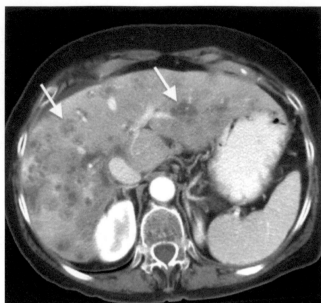

(A) Contrast-enhanced CT in portal venous phase of the liver shows a nodular liver with areas of capsular retraction and hypodense areas of scarring or fibrosis (*arrows*). **(B)** Contrast-enhanced computed tomography in portal venous phase of the liver four years prior to initiation of therapy shows multiple hypodense liver lesions (*arrows*).

■ **Differential Diagnosis**

- **Pseudocirrhosis from treated liver metastasis:** The liver can have a nodular contour after treatment from several types of carcinoma mimicking cirrhosis. Identification of the hypodense metastatic lesions and comparison with historical studies is important.
- *Hepatic cirrhosis:* Occurs in the setting of hepatitis viral infection, alcohol use, or it can be idiopathic. The hepatic nodularity can mimic pseudocirrhosis.
- *Chronic Budd-Chiari syndrome:* Occurs from hepatic venous thrombosis; areas that are well drained tend to hypertrophy producing asymmetric hepatic hypertrophy. Identification of the thrombosed veins and venous collaterals is supportive.
- *Chronic portal vein thrombosis:* Can produce asymmetric hepatic hypertrophy due to areas that are perfused by the portal vein undergoing hypertrophy. Identification of the thrombosed portal vein and cavernous transformation is important.

■ **Essential Facts**

- There is hepatic volume loss with a nodular hepatic contour and variable degrees of caudate hypertrophy.
- Areas of capsular retraction due to chemotherapy or nodular regenerative hyperplasia in the absence of bridging fibrosis.

- A desmoplastic reaction in response to infiltrating tumor can also produce similar imaging findings.
- Treated metastasis from breast, lung, colon, and carcinoid tumor can produce a nodular hepatic contour that mimics cirrhosis.

■ **Other Imaging Findings**

- Magnetic resonance imaging can be useful in evaluating for metastatic lesions, particularly to exclude fatty infiltration, and, in some cases, hepatocellular carcinoma.
- In some cases, liver biopsy may be needed to establish the diagnosis.

✓ **Pearls and ✗ Pitfalls**

✓ Pseudocirrhosis occurs in patients with treated metastatic carcinoma, particularly breast cancer.
✓ It can mimic conventional hepatic cirrhosis.
✓ Patients may develop portal hypertension.
✓ Up to 50% of patients with treated metastatic breast cancer can develop pseudocirrhosis.
✗ It is important to obtain proper history as its imaging features can mimic chronic liver disease and cirrhosis.
✗ It is important to evaluate the hypodense lesions as partially treated metastasis may progress and can be masked by the areas of scarring.

Case 3

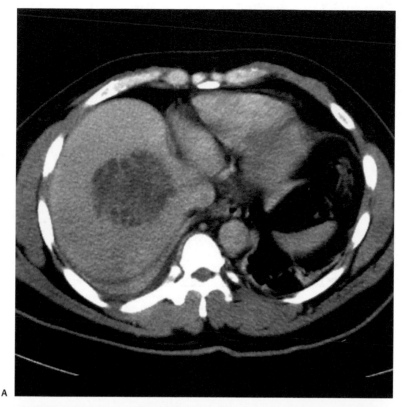

A

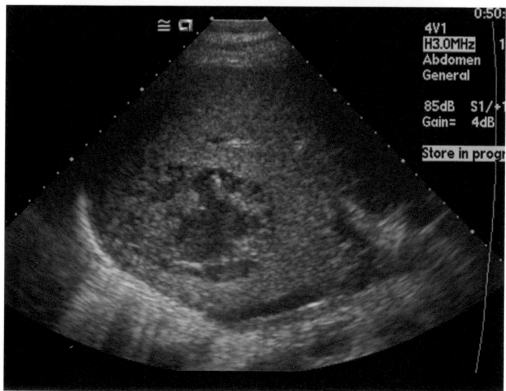

B

■ Clinical Presentation

A 55-year-old male presents with right upper quadrant pain and fever following a bout of diverticulitis.

■ Imaging Findings

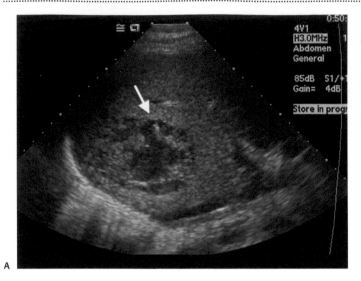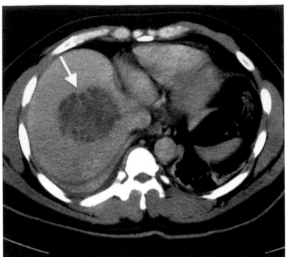

(A) Ultrasound of the right hepatic lobe shows a hypoechoic right hepatic mass with peripheral nodularity (*arrow*). **(B)** Contrast-enhanced computed tomography (CT) in portal venous phase of the liver shows hypovascular lesion consisting of a cluster of multiple near-low-attenuating lesions (*arrow*).

■ Differential Diagnosis

- **Hepatic abscess:** Areas of infected liver that have undergone necrosis. CT demonstrates multiple low-level attenuating lesions with wall enhancement and perfusion abnormality.
- *Hepatic metastasis:* Metastases, most notably from adenocarcinoma, can mimic hepatic abscess as they can undergo necrosis.
- *Multilocular hepatic cyst:* Multiple coalescent hepatic cysts are a benign entity with well-defined thin wall cysts containing fluid.
- *Echinococcal cyst:* Hydatid cystic disease in the liver results from infection with the larval stage of echinococcosis.

■ Essential Facts

- Hepatic abscesses consist of infected necrotic hepatic parenchyma that has undergone liquefaction.
- Early hepatic abscesses that have not undergone necrosis can be hard to detect and may manifest as areas of heterogeneous perfusion surrounding small subtle areas of necrosis.
- At CT in the setting of pyogenic abscess, there is an aggregation of multiple small abscesses in a localized area to form a larger abscess cavity producing the "cluster sign."
- Hepatic abscess may be associated with a transient hepatic attenuation difference distal to the lesion.

■ Other Imaging Findings

- Magnetic resonance imaging may be able to better delineate the cluster of abscesses as multiple T2 hyperintense lesions with wall enhancement. Hepatic abscesses restrict diffusion.
- Hepatic abscess can have a variable appearance at ultrasound, ranging from hypoechoic with some low-level internal echoes to hyperechoic.

✓ Pearls and ✗ Pitfalls

- ✓ Pyogenic hepatic abscesses are mostly due to anaerobic infection.
- ✓ The abscess may have to be drained for treatment.
- ✗ Necrotic metastasis can mimic hepatic abscess.
- ✗ Hepatic abscess may not contain gas.

Case 4

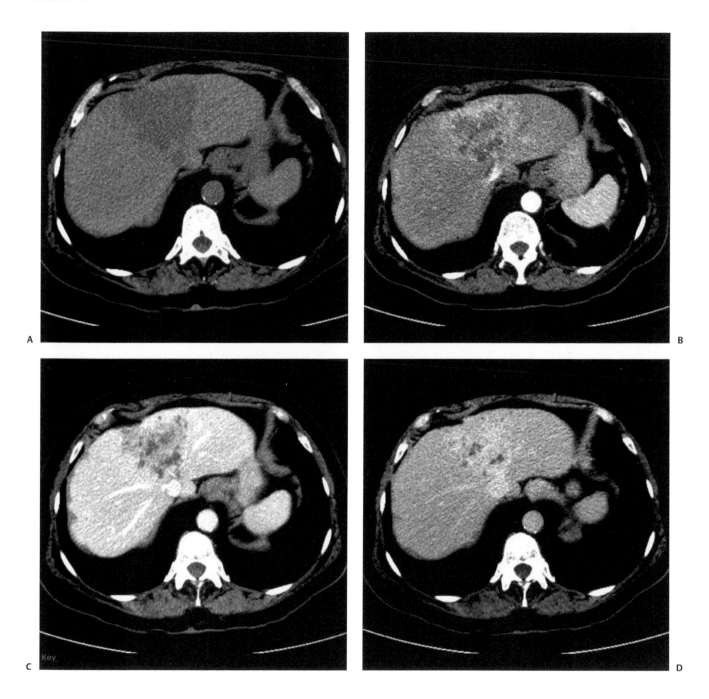

A

B

C

Key

D

■ Clinical Presentation

A 69-year-old female with work-up of an incidentally detected hepatic mass undergoes multiphasic computed tomography (CT).

■ Imaging Findings

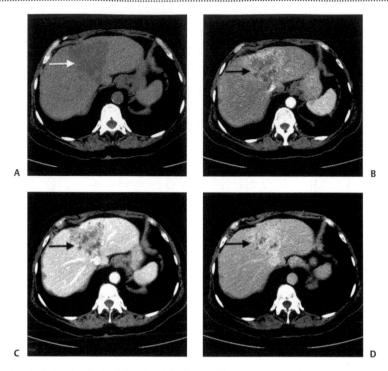

(A) Unenhanced CT shows a wedge-shaped lesion in the left lobe of the liver with an area of capsular retraction near its periphery (*arrow*). **(B)** Arterial phase CT shows ill-defined enhancement of the lesion, mostly along its periphery, with heterogeneous central enhancement (*arrow*). **(C)** Portal phase CT show the mass with multiple hypodense areas to be hypoattenuating to liver parenchyma (*arrow*). **(D)** Delayed phase CT shows contrast retention in the lesion in relation to the background liver (*arrow*).

■ Differential Diagnosis

- **Cholangiocarcinoma:** A primary carcinoma of the biliary tree that can affect the intra- or extrahepatic biliary tree. It can produce focal biliary obstruction distal to the mass.
- *Hepatic metastasis:* Some scirrhous metastatic lesions can produce similar imaging findings. However, metastatic disease tends to have multiple lesions and a known extrahepatic primary.

■ Essential Facts

- Cholangiocarcinoma has three predominant growth patterns (mass-forming, periductal infiltrating, and intraductal type).
- The mass-forming lesions present as solid hepatic masses that are hypoattenuating on noncontrast CT, show peripheral arterial enhancement, and tend to retain contrast on delayed phase CT due to the fibrotic nature of the lesion.
- The periductal infiltrating type is characterized by growth along a dilated or narrowed bile duct without mass formation and manifests as an elongated, spiculated, or branchlike lesion.
- The intraductal type grows slowly and can manifest as diffuse marked duct ectasia with a grossly visible papillary mass.
- The Bismuth-Corlette classification is used to classify hepatic hilar cholangiocarcinoma for resectability.

■ Other Imaging Findings

- Ultrasound may show focally dilated ducts and a mass at the apex, which tends to have a heterogeneous to hyperechoic appearance.
- Magnetic resonance imaging/magnetic resonance cholangiopancreatography is an excellent choice to evaluate the ductal morphology and extent of disease to guide resection.

✓ Pearls and ✗ Pitfalls

✓ Focally dilated ducts, especially with a suggestion of a mass, must be considered suspicious.

✓ Cholangiocarcinoma with a fibrous component shows delayed contrast enhancement that can be used to diagnose the entity.

✓ Cholangiocarcinoma, due to its fibrous nature, can cause capsular retraction that can help differentiate it from other hepatic lesions.

✓ Mass-forming cholangiocarcinoma extends via the portal venous system and via lymphatic invasion.

✗ Treated metastasis with fibrosis can mimic cholangiocarcinoma.

✗ Cholangiocarcinoma can spread to the peritoneum. Peritoneal nodules or ascites should be evaluated for possible carcinomatosis when staging patients.

Case 5

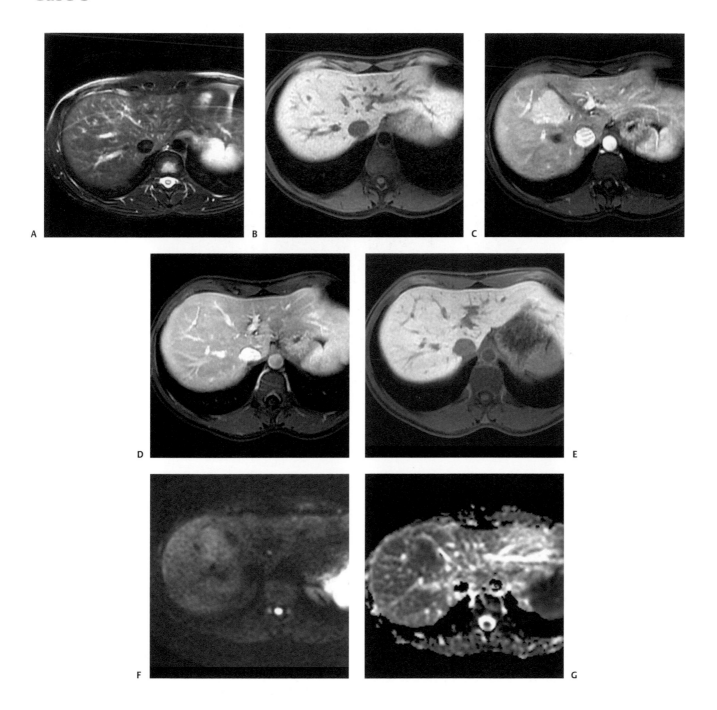

■ **Clinical Presentation**

A 30-year-old female with incidentally detected hepatic mass for further characterization.

■ **Imaging Findings**

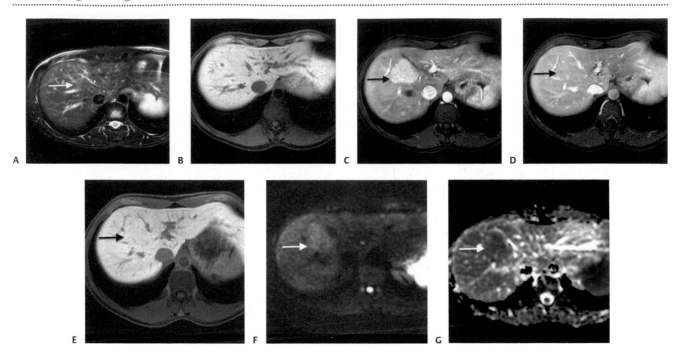

(A) T2 weighted fat-saturated image shows a faint area of increased signal near the middle hepatic vein (*arrow*). **(B)** T1-fast spoiled gradient echo (FSPGR) precontrast image shows no evident abnormality in the area. **(C)** T1-FSPGR with contrast, arterial phase (hepatobiliary contrast agent), shows a hypervascular lesion in segment 8 of the liver (*arrow*). **(D)** T1-FSPGR with contrast, venous phase, shows the lesion is isointense to liver (*arrow*). **(E)** T1-FSPGR with contrast, one-hour delay, shows accumulation of contrast agent in the lesion as it is isointense to liver (*arrow*). **(F)** Diffusion weighted imaging (*b* = 800) shows faint area of increased signal near the middle hepatic vein (*arrow*). **(G)** Apparent diffusion coefficient map shows the abnormality of mild restricted diffusion (*arrow*).

■ **Differential Diagnosis**

- **Focal nodular hyperplasia (FNH):** Benign regenerative hepatic lesion with no known malignant potential formed from hyperplastic growth of normal hepatocytes but malformed biliary drainage.
- *Hepatic adenoma:* Benign hepatic lesion that has several subtypes, some of which can be a precursor for carcinoma. These lesions do not accumulate a hepatic specific agent.
- *Hepatocellular carcinoma:* Primary hepatic malignancy that arises most commonly in the setting of chronic liver disease. Hypervascular on arterial phase, these lesions wash out on delayed imaging.
- *Hypervascular metastasis:* Metastatic disease from renal, thyroid, neuroendocrine, and some adenocarcinomas. These lesions are usually hyperintense on T2 imaging and washout on delayed imaging.

■ **Essential Facts**

- FNH is a benign hyperplastic hepatic lesion with absent biliary drainage.
- FNH blood supply is from the hepatic artery and drainage is via the hepatic veins. FNH lesions are uniformly hypervascular and are isointense to liver on portal and delayed phases of imaging.

- They accumulate hepatobiliary-specific contrast agents, and this feature is useful to confirm the diagnosis.
- Larger lesions can have a central T2-hyperintense scar.

■ **Other Imaging Findings**

- On computed tomography, FNH shows brisk arterial enhancement and no washout on portal venous or delayed phases. The lesions tend to have a lobular margin.
- Ultrasound may not detect FNH as they can appear similar to background liver. They can sometimes depict the central artery on color or power Doppler.

✓ **Pearls and** ✗ **Pitfalls**

- ✓ Classic FNH has a T2-hyperintense central scar and central artery.
- ✓ FNH lesions can have a lobular contour and do not washout on delayed imaging using a hepatobilary agent.
- ✗ Atypical FNH lacks the central scar and central artery.
- ✗ FNH can show mild restricted diffusion and should not be mistaken for a malignant lesion.
- ✗ FNH may rarely contain intralesional fat.

Case 6

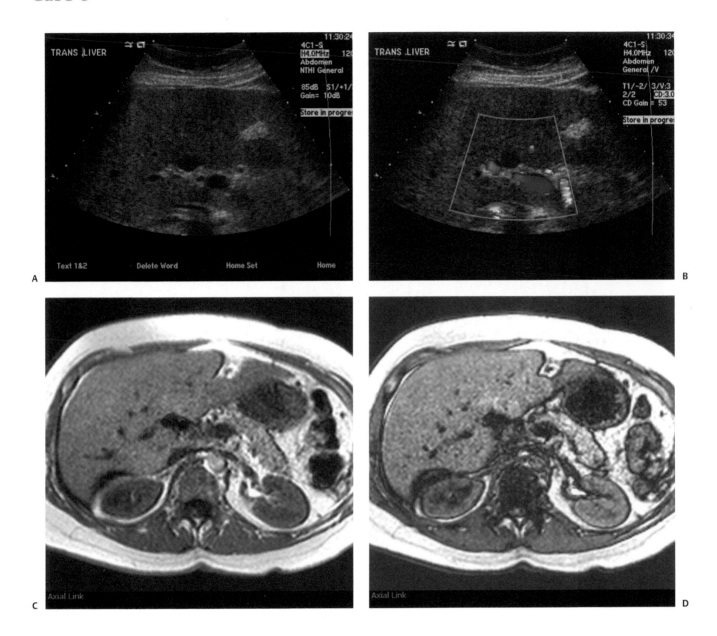

■ **Clinical Presentation**

A 45-year-old female with elevated liver function tests undergoes ultrasound.

■ Imaging Findings

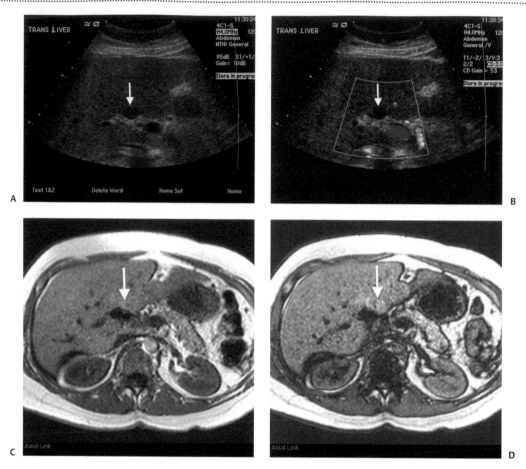

(A) Ultrasound of the liver shows a focal hypoechoic lesion (*arrow*); the background liver parenchyma is mildly hyperechoic. **(B)** Color Doppler image shows no flow in the lesion, which is adjacent to the portal vein (*arrow*). **(C)** T1-fast spoiled gradient echo (FSPGR) in-phase shows the lesion to be nearly isointense to liver (*arrow*). **(D)** T1-FSPGR-out of-phase shows the lesion to be hyperintense to liver (*arrow*).

■ Differential Diagnosis

- **Focal fatty sparing (FFS):** Geographic areas in the liver near the gallbladder fossa or near the portal vein are typical areas where fat is not deposited.
- *Hepatic adenoma:* Hepatic lesion that is rounded and can contain intralesional fat.

■ Essential Facts

- FFS typically occurs adjacent to the portal vein, near the gallbladder fossa, near the hepatic fissures, and in the subcapsular area.
- They are typically hypoechoic on ultrasound and show signal preservation in/out of phase T1-FSPGR imaging compared with the background liver.

■ Other Imaging Findings

- On computed tomography, FFS may be hyperattenuating to the liver in a geographic pattern in one of the usual locations.
- This can produce areas of differential perfusion on computed tomography.

✓ Pearls and ✗ Pitfalls

- ✓ Areas of FFS can have geographic borders and lack mass effect.
- ✓ There is no distortion of vessels as they course through the area of FFS.
- ✓ There can be regional perfusion changes about the area of FFS.
- ✗ FFS may have a nodular appearance and may mimic a lesion.

Case 7

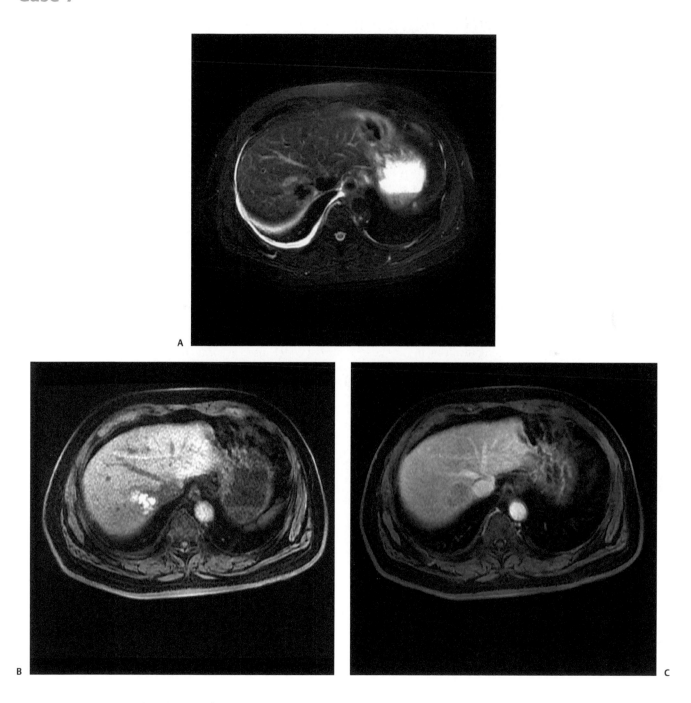

A

B

C

■ Clinical Presentation

A 76-year-old-male with liver lesion for work-up.

■ Imaging Findings

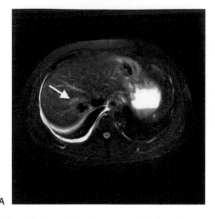 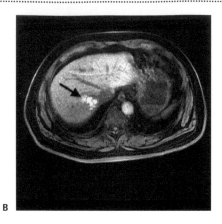 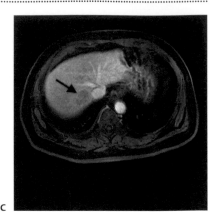

A   B   C

(A) Axial T2-weighted imaging of the liver shows a mildly T2-hyperintense lesion near the right hepatic vein with central T2-hypointensity (*arrow*). **(B)** Axial T1–fast spoiled gradient echo (FSPGR) precontrast shows the lesion to be markedly hyperintense compared to liver (*arrow*). **(C)** Axial T1-FSPGR postcontrast shows the lesion as hypointense compared to liver (*arrow*).

■ Differential Diagnosis

• ***Melanoma metastasis:*** Melanin from metastatic melanoma produces T1 shortening resulting in T1 hyperintensity.
• *Focal hemorrhage:* Hemorrhage can also produce T1 hyperintensity.
• *Hepatocellular carcinoma:* Primary liver cancer can undergo hemorrhage and produce T1 hyperintensity.

■ Essential Facts

• Metastatic melanoma can produce T1-hyperintense metastatic deposits in the liver.
• Other compounds can cause T1 shortening in the liver including fat, blood products from hemorrhage, copper, melanin, and highly concentrated proteins. Several lesions such as hepatocellular carcinoma and dysplastic nodules can also be T1-hyperintense.

■ Other Imaging Findings

• F18–fluorodeoxyglucose positron emission tomography is a widely used accurate modality in the evaluation of metastatic disease from melanoma. The lesions are easily detected as they are very fluorodeoxyglucose avid.

✓ Pearls and ✗ Pitfalls

✓ Fat-suppressed T1-FSPGR images help detect fatty masses.
✓ Subtraction T1-FSPGR postcontrast images can help detect enhancement in inherently T1-hyperintense masses.
✗ Many lesions can appear T1-hyperintense to liver in the setting of diffuse fatty infiltration as the background liver loses signal in fat suppressed T1-FSPGR images.

Case 8

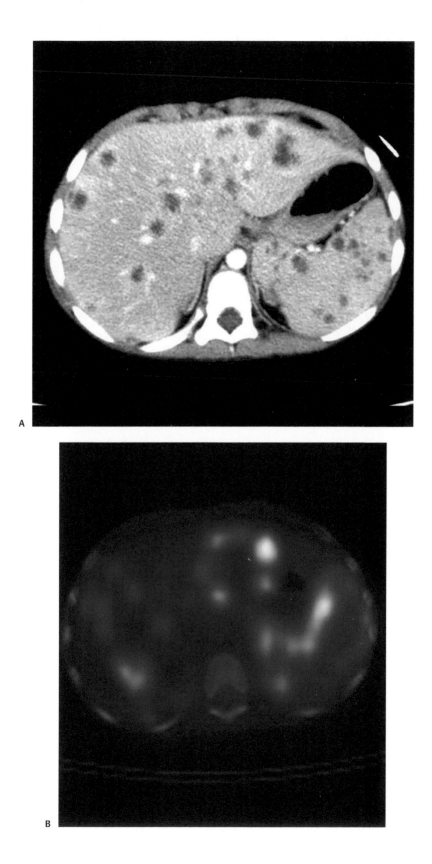

A

B

■ Clinical Presentation

An 8-year-old male with acute lymphocytic leukemia on therapy presents with new liver and splenic lesions.

■ **Imaging Findings**

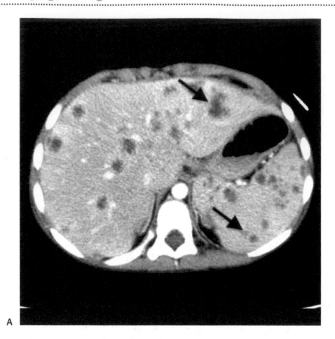
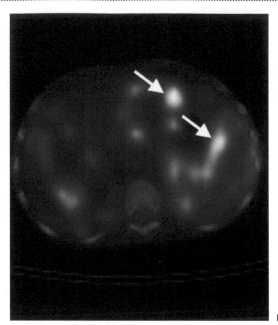

(A) Contrast-enhanced computed tomography (CT) shows numerous hepatic and splenic hypodense lesions. The liver lesions have an enhancing wall (*arrows*).
(B) F18–fluorodeoxyglucose (FDG) positron emission tomography/CT shows numerous foci of avid FDG activity in the liver and spleen (*arrows*).

■ **Differential Diagnosis**

• ***Disseminated fungal infection with abscess:***
Multiple lesions in the liver and spleen in an immunocompromised patient that appear soon after induction of chemotherapy should raise the suspicion for infection.
• *Metastatic disease:* Metastatic disease can be difficult to discriminate from fungal abscesses.
• *Sarcoidosis:* Patients with sarcoid frequently have lung findings and other clinical findings.

■ **Essential Facts**

• In the immunocompromised pediatric patient, concurrent hepatic and splenic lesions usually represent microabscesses resulting from disseminated fungal disease.
• Early identification is important for therapy.

■ **Other Imaging Findings**

• The ultrasound will show multiple hypoechoic lesions. They may have low-level internal echoes depending on the stage of the abscess formation.

✓ **Pearls and** ✗ **Pitfalls**

✓ Multiple splenic and hepatic lesions that develop in an immunocompromised patient should raise the suspicion for multiple abscesses.
✓ Biopsy or aspiration of the lesions may be necessary to rule out alternatives such as metastatic disease and to determine the microorganism.
✗ Infectious processes can show marked F18-FDG avidity.

Case 9

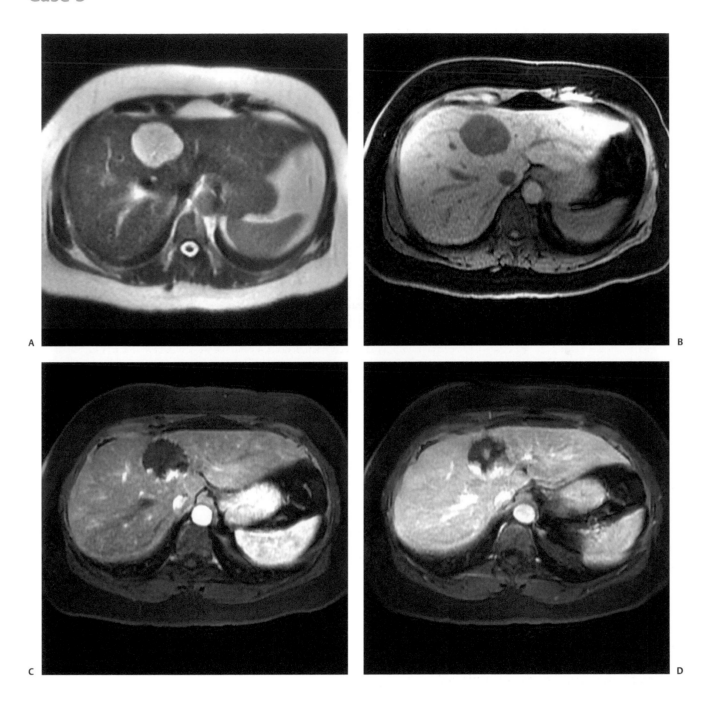

A

B

C

D

■ **Clinical Presentation**

A 64-year-old female with hepatic mass for further evaluation.

■ **Imaging Findings**

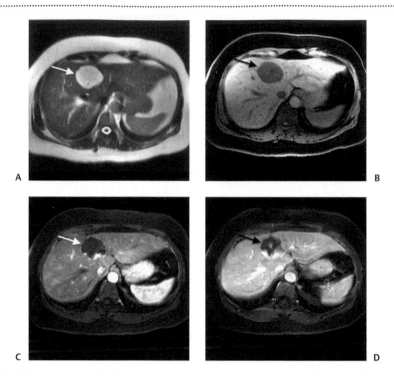

(A) Axial T2-weighted image (WI) of the liver shows a T2-hyperintense lesion in the liver (*arrow*). **(B)** Axial T1-fast spoiled gradient echo (FSPGR) precontrast shows the hypointense lesion in the liver (*arrow*). **(C)** Axial T1-FSPGR postcontrast, arterial phase, shows peripheral nodular discontinuous enhancement of the lesion (*arrow*). **(D)** Axial T1-FSPGR postcontrast, venous phase, shows progressive centripetal fill-in of the lesion with contrast (*arrow*).

■ **Differential Diagnosis**

- ***Hemangioma:*** Hemangiomas are the second most common benign liver lesion after hepatic cysts with a prevalence of 8.6%. They are hypervascular and show the typical enhancement pattern with nodularity and progression from peripheral to central.
- *Hepatic metastasis:* The liver is a frequent site for metastasis from abdominal, lung, and breast malignancies. Metastatic disease lacks the classic nodular peripheral enhancement of hemangiomas.
- *Epithelioid hemangioendothelioma:* A rare hypervascular liver tumor that has a typical ring morphology on T2-WI.

■ **Essential Facts**

- Hemangiomas are benign hepatic lesions that can be diagnosed on multiphasic contrast-enhanced magnetic resonance imaging (MRI) by the characteristic pattern of peripheral nodular discontinuous enhancement at the hepatic arterial phase with progressive centripetal fill-in.
- The lesions are characteristically T2 hyperintense.
- Some small hemangiomas appear as solid-enhancing lesions but do not washout.
- Sclerosed hemangiomas can have variable rates of enhancement, may have calcification, and can pose a diagnostic dilemma in a patient with a suspected malignancy.

■ **Other Imaging Findings**

- Ultrasound shows hemangiomas typically as hyperechoic masses.
- When the liver has fatty infiltration or has increased background echogenicity, they can present as hypoechoic masses.
- On computed tomography (CT), hemangiomas attenuate similar to blood pool on noncontrast images, show peripheral nodular enhancement, and progressively fill in.

✓ **Pearls and ✗ Pitfalls**

- ✓ Hemangiomas can have variable rates of contrast fill-in and, therefore, delayed imaging is helpful to distinguish them from alternatives such as metastatic disease.
- ✗ Small hypervascular metastasis may mimic a flash-filling hemangioma on a single-phase exam.
- ✗ Sclerosing hepatic hemangioma can have overlapping imaging features with malignant entities such as cholangiocarcinoma on T2-WI and postcontrast T1-WI.

Case 10

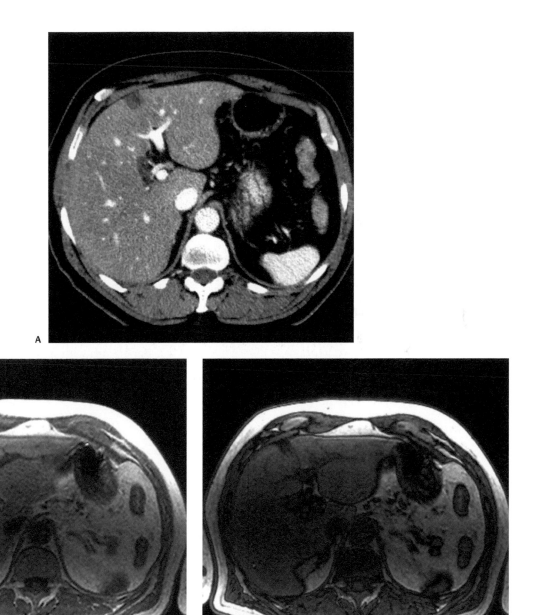

■ Clinical Presentation

A 78-year-old male with a known malignancy with work-up of liver lesion.

■ **Imaging Findings**

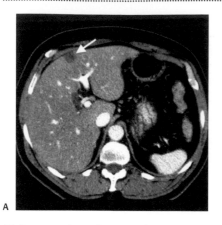 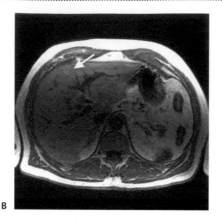 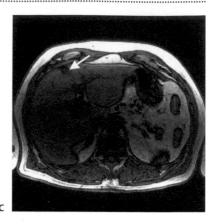

(A) Contrast-enhanced computed tomography (CT) shows focal hypodense lesion near the falciform ligament (*arrow*). **(B)** T1-fast spoiled gradient echo (FSPGR) in-phase shows the lesion to be nearly isointense to liver (*arrow*). **(C)** T1-FSPGR out-of-phase shows the lesion to be hypointense to liver, losing signal (*arrow*).

■ **Differential Diagnosis**

- ***Focal fatty infiltration:*** A common finding that is incidentally discovered in typical locations.
- *Metastasis:* The liver is a common site for metastatic disease from malignancies originating from the abdomen, lung, and breast. It tends to be rounded, multiple, and occur in the right hepatic lobe, possibly due to increased blood flow compared with the left.

■ **Essential Facts**

- Focal fatty deposition has a predilection for several regions including the medial segment of the left lobe of the liver adjacent to the falciform ligament, near the gallbladder fossa, the anterior portion of the caudate, and the posterior portion of segment IV.
- It tends to be geographic, and vessels pass through the region without compression or displacement.

■ **Other Imaging Findings**

- On sonography, focal fat is imaged as a hyperechoic geographic area with vessels coursing through it.
- Focal fat is most commonly detected near the portal vein.

✓ **Pearls and ✗ Pitfalls**

- ✓ Focal fat can mimic a hypoattenuating lesion on single-phase CT.
- ✓ Focal fat tends to have a nonspherical border and does not have regional mass effect.
- ✓ Atypical patterns include multinodular, mass-like, and perivascular deposition that can mimic malignancies.
- ✗ Fat-containing lesions such as hepatocellular carcinoma and hepatic adenoma may be mistaken for focal fatty infiltration. In these cases, contrast enhancement pattern as well as vascular compression or displacement may help differentiate these entities from focal fat.

Case 11

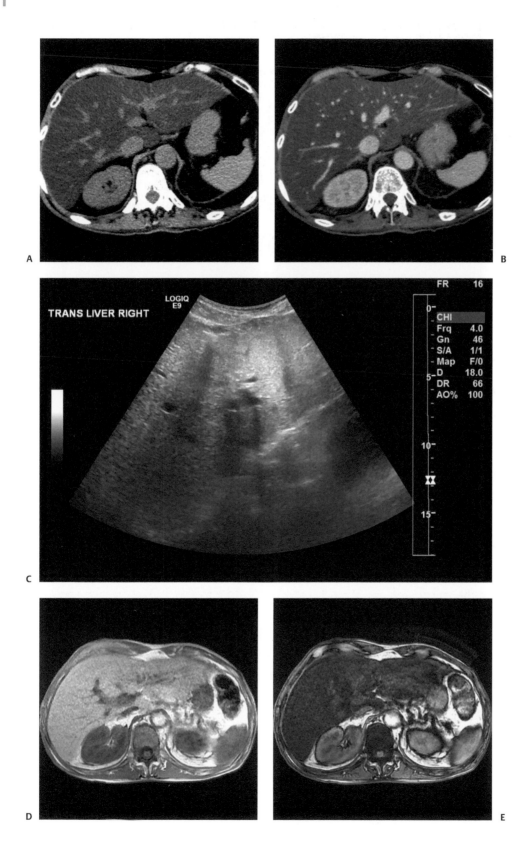

■ Clinical Presentation

A 54-year-old male with elevated liver enzymes for further evaluation.

■ Imaging Findings

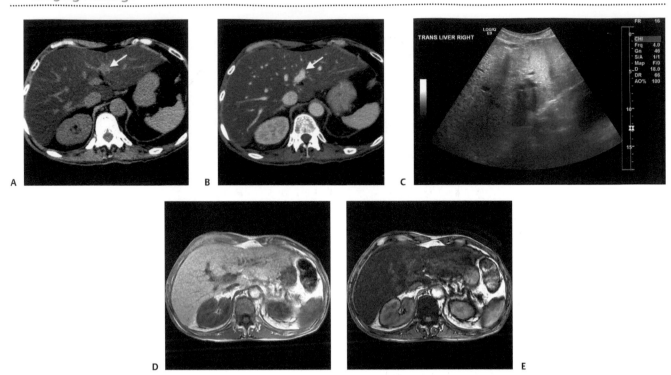

(A) Noncontrast computed tomography (CT) shows the hepatic parenchyma as hypodense compared with the vessels (*arrow*). **(B)** Contrast-enhanced CT shows the hepatic parenchyma hypodense to the spleen (*arrow*). **(C)** Ultrasound of the liver shows echogenic hepatic parenchyma that attenuates the sound beam. **(D, E)** T1-fast spoiled gradient echo (FSPGR) in/opposed phase shows signal loss in the liver indicating hepatic steatosis.

■ Differential Diagnosis

- ***Hepatic steatosis:*** Diffuse hepatic steatosis can be due to metabolic causes and medications, among other processes.
- *Infiltrative process:* Some infiltrative processes can mimic hepatic steatosis.

■ Essential Facts

- Nonalcoholic fatty liver disease is the most common cause of chronic liver disease and affects nearly one-third of the U.S. population.
- Chronic hepatic steatosis can result in nonalcoholic steatohepatitis, which can lead to chronic liver disease, cirrhosis, and the development of hepatocellular carcinoma.
- CT is able to detect moderate to severe fatty infiltration but is unable to quantify it.
- Magnetic resonance imaging (MRI) is able to detect and quantify hepatic fatty infiltration. The liver can be enlarged and show areas of asymmetric hypertrophy.

■ Other Imaging Findings

- On ultrasound, diffuse hepatic steatosis results in a very echogenic liver.
- The vessels are obscured and there is poor beam penetration, which can limit its utility.

✓ Pearls and ✗ Pitfalls

- ✓ MRI with in/opposed phase imaging can be used to detect hepatic steatosis. Iterative decomposition of water and fat with echo asymmetry and the least-squares estimation (IDEAL) can be employed to calculate fat percentages.
- ✓ CT can detect moderate to severe steatosis using thresholds of < 40 HU attenuation of liver or a difference in attenuation between liver and spleen of more than −10 HU on unenhanced CT.
- ✗ Hepatic lesions can easily be obscured in a fatty liver on CT as the difference in attenuation between the lesion and the background liver is lost.

Case 12

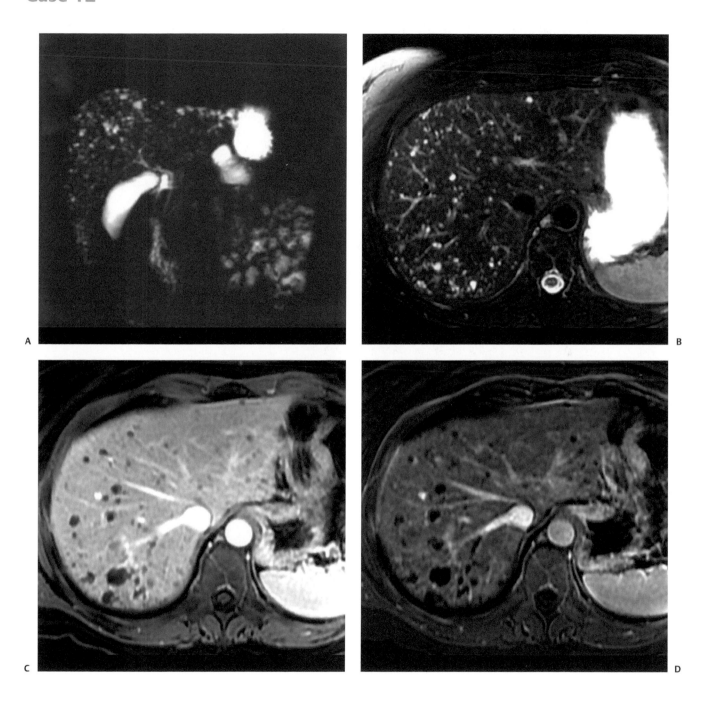

■ Clinical Presentation

A 57-year-old female with multiple liver lesions for further evaluation with magnetic resonance imaging.

■ Imaging Findings

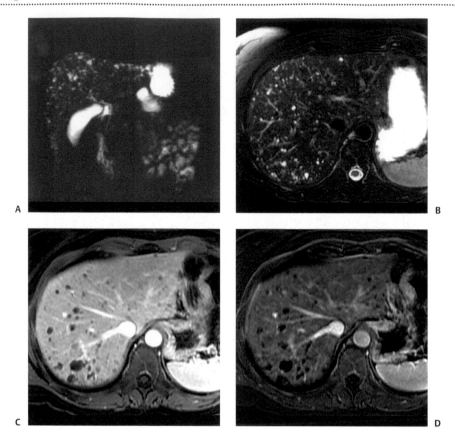

(A) Coronal thick slab magnetic resonance cholangiopancreatography showing innumerable small T2-hyperintense lesions in the liver. Note the biliary tree is normal. **(B)** Axial T2-weighted imaging with fat saturation shows multiple small lesions, some irregular in shape but with well-defined margins. **(C)** Axial T1-fast spoiled gradient echo (FSPGR) + C shows the lesions are well defined, some with irregular margins but without enhancement. **(D)** Axial T1-FSPGR + C subtraction sequence shows the lesions do not enhance.

■ Differential Diagnosis

- **Biliary hamartomas:** Benign hepatic lesions that mimic cysts but are histologically unique. They tend to have a similar size throughout the liver and can be quite numerous.
- *Hepatic cysts:* Hepatic cysts are the most common benign hepatic lesion and have a prevalence of about 15%. They have well-defined margins and can be of varying size.

■ Essential Facts

- Biliary hamartomas are benign lesions that are the result of ductal plate malformations.
- When multiple, they are known by the eponym Von Meyenburg complexes.
- They vary in size from 1 to 15 mm.

■ Other Imaging Findings

- On ultrasound, the numerous echogenic wall interfaces can make the liver have a heterogeneous appearance, and individual cystic areas may not be resolved if they are numerous.
- On computed tomography, the lesions are small, well-defined, and do not enhance. Their small size can limit measurement of Hounsfield units and can mimic small metastases or abscesses.

✓ Pearls and ✗ Pitfalls

- ✓ Biliary hamartomas are easily detected using a T2-weighted sequence, but contrast is required to make sure the lesions do not enhance.
- ✓ Biliary hamartomas do not communicate with the biliary tree and hence do not accumulate hepatobiliary-specific contrast agents.
- ✗ Biliary hamartomas are associated with cholangiocarcinoma, like other ductal plate abnormalities.

Case 13

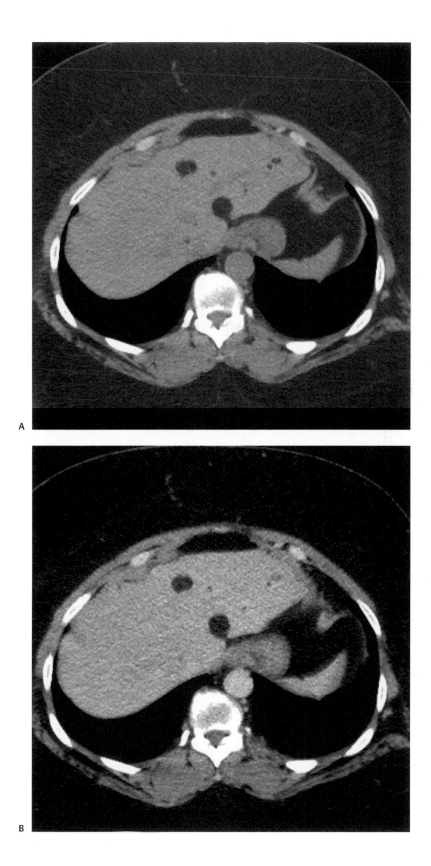

■ Clinical Presentation

A 42-year-old female with multiple hepatic lesions for further characterization.

■ **Imaging Findings**

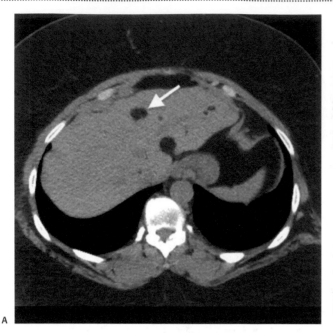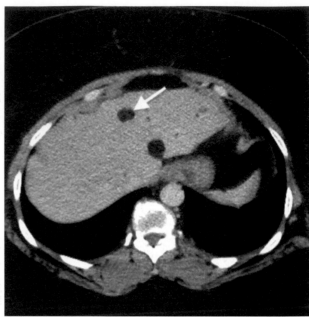

A   B

(A) Unenhanced computed tomography (CT) of the liver shows several fat-attenuating lesions in the left hepatic lobe (*arrow*). **(B)** Contrast-enhanced CT of the liver shows no evident enhancement in the lesions (*arrow*).

■ **Differential Diagnosis**

- ***Hepatic angiomyolipoma (HAML):*** A benign hepatic lesion that contains variable amounts of fat. It is easily detected on CT as a fatty mass and is easier to characterize when found in conjunction with tuberous sclerosis complex.
- *Hepatic adenoma:* A benign lesion that can be hypervascular on arterial phase and show varying degrees of washout. Hepatic adenoma can contain varying amounts tumoral fat, tends to occur in females, and is associated with contraceptive use.
- *Hepatocellular carcinoma:* Well-differentiated hepatocellular carcinoma can contain fat but occurs in patients in the setting of chronic liver disease and cirrhosis.

■ **Essential Facts**

- HAML is a rare, benign mesenchymal neoplasm that consists of varying numbers of smooth muscle cells, thick-walled blood vessels, and mature adipose tissue.
- HAML can occur in patients with or without tuberous sclerosis complex.
- Lesions that contain mature fat and lack a capsule can be identified as HAML. Lesions that are fat-deficient HAML are harder to diagnose and may require a biopsy.

■ **Other Imaging Findings**

- Fat-containing lesions lose signal on fat-saturated sequences and are hyperintense on nonfat-saturated T1 images.
- If the lesion contains fat admixed with other elements, the lesion will lose signal on opposed-phase imaging.

✓ **Pearls and ✗ Pitfalls**

- ✓ HAML can have a central draining vein that drains to the hepatic vein.
- ✓ Fat-containing HAML is characterized by the presence of mature fat in the lesion.
- ✗ Fat-deficient HAML can show arterial enhancement and washout.
- ✗ In the setting of cirrhosis or chronic viral hepatitis, hepatocellular carcinoma should be considered.

Case 14

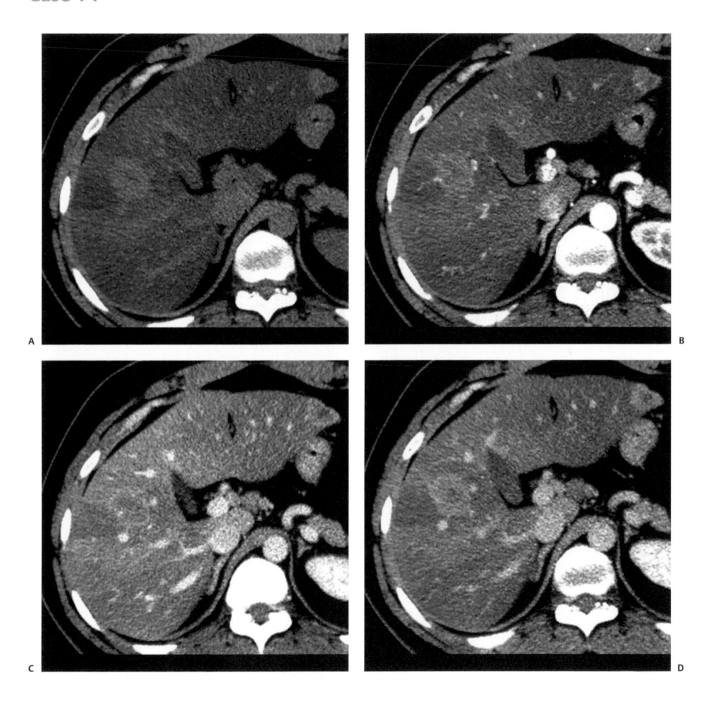

■ **Clinical Presentation**

A 38-year-old male with multiple hepatic lesions for further characterization.

■ **Imaging Findings**

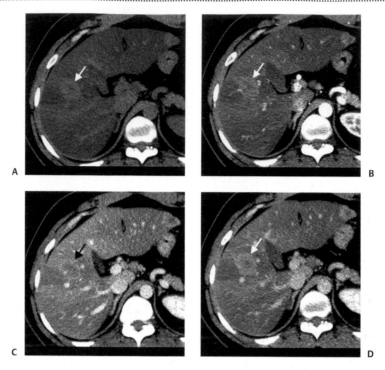

(A) Unenhanced computed tomography (CT) of the liver shows a hyperattenuating lesion in the right hepatic lobe in the setting of fatty infiltration (*arrow*). Note the second lesion in the left lateral segment. **(B)** Contrast-enhanced CT, arterial phase, of the liver shows mild enhancement of the lesion (*arrow*). **(C)** Contrast-enhanced CT, portal venous phase, shows the lesion is hypointense to liver (*arrow*). **(D)** Delayed phase CT shows the lesion to be mildly hyperdense to liver (*arrow*).

■ **Differential Diagnosis**

- **Hepatic lymphoma:** Primary hepatic lymphoma is a rare malignant lesion of the liver. Biopsy may be needed to diagnose the entity.
- *Hepatic adenoma:* A benign lesion that can be hypervascular on arterial phase and show varying degrees of washout. They can contain varying amounts of fat or lipid. They tend to occur in females and are associated with contraceptive use.
- *Hepatocellular carcinoma:* Primary hepatic malignancy that is typically hypervascular at the arterial phase and shows portal venous or delayed washout. It is associated with chronic liver disease and cirrhosis.

■ **Essential Facts**

- Hepatic lymphoma can be either primary or secondary. In primary lymphoma, the disease is confined to the liver. Hepatic involvement is seen in up to 50% of the cases in secondary lymphoma at autopsy.
- The pattern of involvement is variable and can present as a solitary hepatic mass; multifocal disease with lesions measuring 1 to 5 cm, as in this case; and diffuse hepatic infiltration.

- On CT, lymphomatous nodules commonly have soft tissue attenuation but enhance to a lesser degree than the liver parenchyma on arterial, portal venous, and delayed phase images.
- The lesions may demonstrate hemorrhage, necrosis, or a rim-enhancement pattern. Calcification is rare in the absence of treatment.
- On magnetic resonance imaging, a central T2-hyperintense "target" area can be present, shown on CT as a central hypodense area.

■ **Other Imaging Findings**

- Hepatic lymphoma can present as multiple hypoechoic lesions on ultrasound and typically mimics metastatic disease.

✓ **Pearls and** ✗ **Pitfalls**

- ✓ Hepatic lymphoma can have several imaging presentations including solitary, multifocal, and infiltrative.
- ✓ Biopsy may be indicated to establish diagnosis in the absence of known history of lymphoma.
- ✗ Diffuse involvement can mimic hepatic steatosis.

Case 15

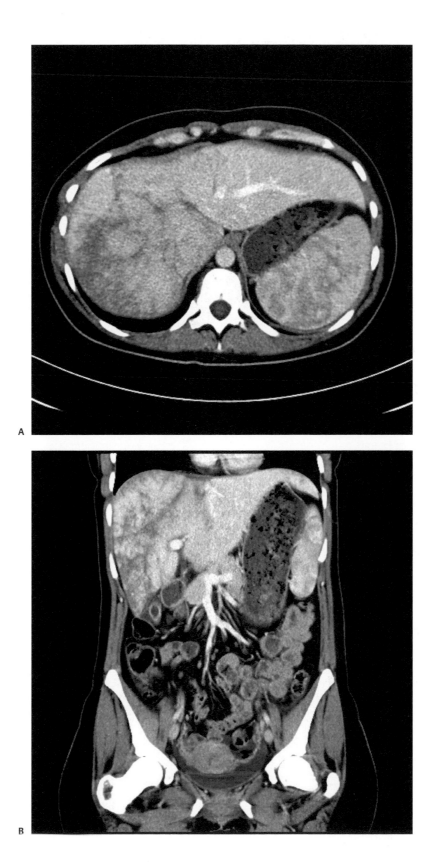

A

B

■ Clinical Presentation

A 37-year-old female with elevated liver enzymes undergoes contrast-enhanced computed tomography (CT) of the liver.

■ **Imaging Findings**

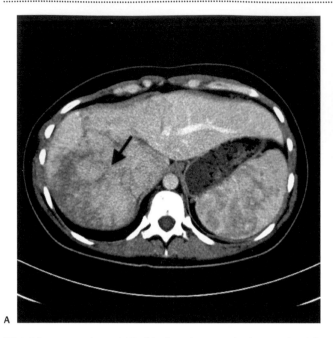 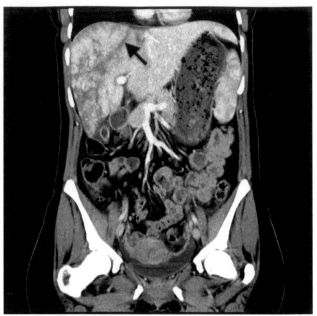

(A) Axial contrast-enhanced CT of the liver shows patchy decreased peripheral enhancement of the liver (*arrow*). **(B)** Coronal contrast-enhanced CT of the liver shows thrombosis of the right hepatic vein (*arrow*).

■ **Differential Diagnosis**

- *Hepatic venous occlusion:* Hepatic venous occlusion can be acute, chronic, or asymptomatic. Acutely, it can present with pain, ascites, and liver enlargement.
- *Portal venous occlusion:* Portal venous occlusion can be secondary to either malignant or benign causes. Most cases are asymptomatic; over time, collateral venous supply develops.

■ **Essential Facts**

- Primary Budd-Chiari syndrome results from hepatic venous outflow occlusion due to thrombus. Secondary results from extrinsic compression.
- Budd-Chiari syndrome can be acute, subacute, or chronic.
- In acute Budd-Chiari syndrome, there is nonfilling of the hepatic vein(s) and patchy, decreased peripheral enhancement caused by portal and sinusoidal stasis. There can be ascites due to increased portal pressure.
- In chronic Budd-Chiari syndrome, venous collaterals develop. There can be caudate hypertrophy and splenomegaly.

■ **Other Imaging Findings**

- Ultrasound findings include absence of flow in the hepatic veins and detection of hepatic venous collaterals along the liver surface.

✓ **Pearls and** ✗ **Pitfalls**

✓ Hepatic venous thrombosis can be easier to identify on coronal images.
✓ Portal venous thrombosis may develop as the result of underlying thrombophilia and poor hepatopetal portal flow due to increased portal pressures.
✗ In chronic Budd-Chiari syndrome, the thrombosed hepatic veins may not be evident and may calcify.
✗ Regenerative nodules can develop in the chronic setting and should be distinguished from hepatocellular carcinoma, which can also develop in the setting of chronic Budd-Chiari syndrome.

Case 16

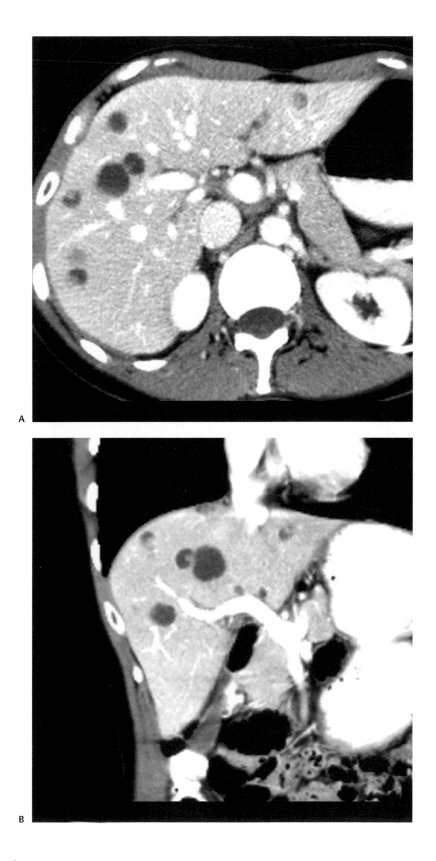

■ Clinical Presentation

A 32-year-old female with history of gastrointestinal stromal tumor.

■ **Imaging Findings**

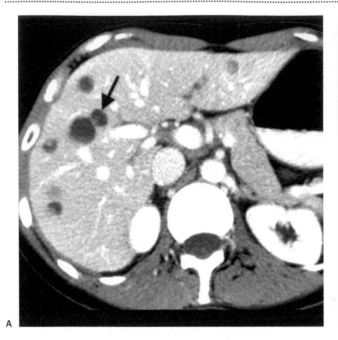 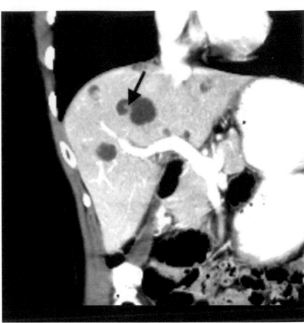

A   B

(A) Axial contrast-enhanced computed tomography (CT) of the liver shows multiple "cystic" lesions with a small mural wall nodule (*arrow*). **(B)** Coronal contrast-enhanced CT of the liver shows the "nearly cystic" lesions in the liver (*arrow*).

■ **Differential Diagnosis**

- **Cystic metastasis:** Cystic metastatic disease is common to several malignancies including gastrointestinal stromal tumors, adenocarcinoma, melanoma, and rarely renal metastasis. They have a less-defined border than hepatic cysts.
- *Hepatic cysts:* Hepatic cysts are the most common benign hepatic lesion and have a prevalence of about 15%. They have well-defined margins and can be of varying size.

■ **Essential Facts**

- Gastrointestinal stromal tumors typically metastasize to the liver and peritoneum.
- Before treatment, the metastases show enhancement on CT.
- Following treatment with a targeted therapy with high specificity for the c-kit protooncogene, the lesions appear "cystlike" and typically decrease in size. When mural nodules (increased attenuation) are present despite total decrease in lesion size, it should be considered tumor progression.

■ **Other Imaging Findings**

- F18–fluorodeoxyglucose positron emission tomography/ CT can be useful as these lesions can have a hypermetabolic wall, unlike cysts.

✓ **Pearls and** ✗ **Pitfalls**

- ✓ Multiphasic CT can be helpful in detecting enhancement in nearly cystic metastasis.
- ✓ Multiplanar imaging is useful in detecting nodules along the superior and inferior walls.
- ✗ Several malignancies can produce cystic metastasis, including germ cell tumors, lung, breast, colon, and sarcomas that can mimic hepatic cysts.
- ✗ Measurement of lesion size may be less accurate than measuring lesion attenuation.

Case 17

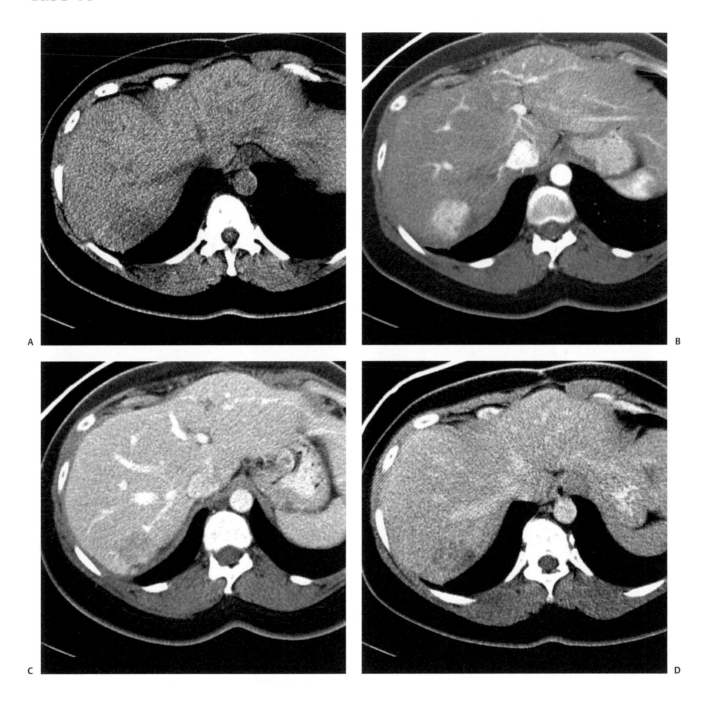

A

B

C

D

■ **Clinical Presentation**

A 36-year-old female with no history of liver disease on oral contraceptives for work-up of a liver lesion.

■ **Imaging Findings**

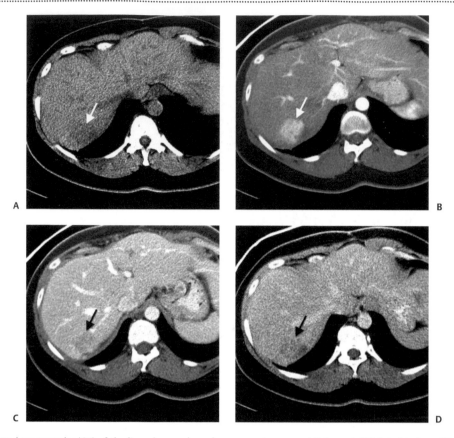

(A) Unenhanced computed tomography (CT) of the liver shows a hypodense mass in segment 7 (*arrow*). **(B)** Arterial phase CT of the liver shows brisk enhancement of the mass (*arrow*). **(C)** Portal venous phase CT shows the mass to be slightly hypoattenuating to liver (*arrow*). **(D)** Delayed phase CT shows the mass hypoattenuating to liver parenchyma (*arrow*).

■ **Differential Diagnosis**

- ***Hepatic adenoma:*** A benign lesion that can be hypervascular on arterial phase and show varying degrees of washout. They can contain varying amounts of fat or lipid. They tend to occur in females and are associated with contraceptive use.
- *Hepatocellular carcinoma (HCC):* Primary hepatic malignancy that is typically hypervascular at the arterial phase and shows portal venous or delayed washout. It is associated with chronic liver disease and cirrhosis.

■ **Essential Facts**

- Hepatocellular adenoma is a rare liver disease with increased incidence in patients on oral contraceptives, anabolic steroids, glycogen storage diseases, and some congenital diseases. There are four histologic subtypes, and the β-catenin-mutated type has a risk of developing HCC. Hepatocellular adenoma can show washout on portal venous or delayed phase imaging and can be difficult to distinguish from HCC. Hepatocellular adenoma can contain tumoral fat or lipid.

■ **Other Imaging Findings**

- Hepatic adenomas can have variable imaging findings on ultrasound as they may undergo hemorrhage.
- Similarly, at CT, they can have a heterogeneous appearance but show similar contrast enhancement as in magnetic resonance imaging.

✓ **Pearls and ✗ Pitfalls**

✓ Large hepatocellular adenomas have an increased risk of hemorrhage.
✓ Hepatocellular adenoma can contain fat.
✗ HCC and hepatocellular adenoma can be difficult to distinguish as both can show washout on delayed imaging.
✗ Certain subtypes of hepatocellular adenoma have an increased risk of HCC development.

Case 18

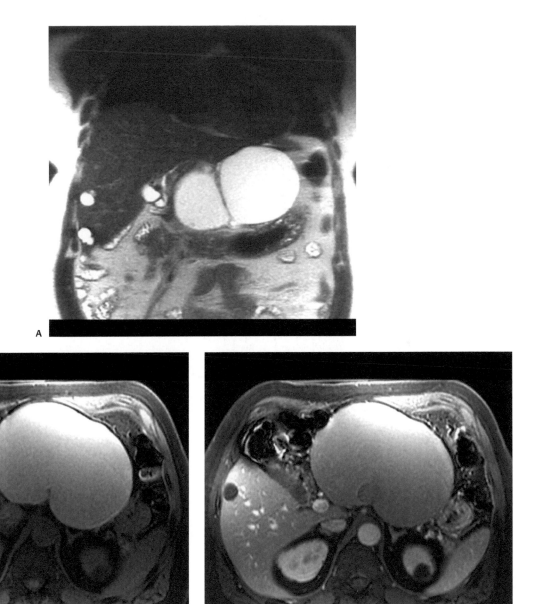

A

B

C

■ **Clinical Presentation**

A 72-year-old female presents with a cystic liver mass.

■ **Imaging Findings**

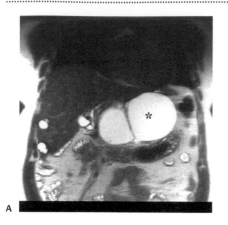 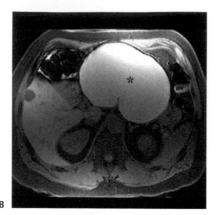 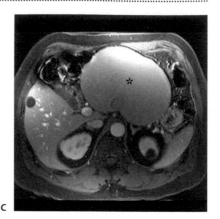

(A) Coronal T2-weighted sequence shows a large, septated, left hepatic cystic lesion (*asterisk*). **(B)** Axial T1-fast spoiled gradient echo (FSPGR) precontrast shows the cystic lesion as T1-hyperintense, indicating hemorrhage or protein content (*asterisk*). **(C)** Axial T1-FSPGR postcontrast shows the cystic lesion has no evident nodular enhancement (*asterisk*).

■ **Differential Diagnosis**

- **Biliary cystadenoma:** A rare benign cystic lesion in the liver. It occurs predominately in middle-aged women.
- *Biliary cystadenocarcinoma:* The malignant neoplasm arises de novo from the biliary tree or malignant transformation of a biliary cystadenoma.
- *Giant biliary hamartoma:* A benign cystic lesion due to malformations of the bile duct plate.

■ **Essential Facts**

- Biliary cystadenoma is a slow-growing cystic neoplasm arising from the bile ducts. It is most common in women with a mean age at presentation of 45 years. The lesions may be unilocular or multilocular.
- Biliary cystadenocarcinoma is considered a malignant transformation of biliary cystadenoma, although de novo cases have been reported. The malignant form should be considered when there are thick walls, nodular enhancement, or malignant features.

■ **Other Imaging Findings**

- The lesion is anechoic, similar to a simple cyst or complex fluid depending on its contents.
- Internal complexity such as septae, nodules, and calcifications can be detected.
- In computed tomography, the lesion may have different attenuation compared with a cyst, depending on its content. Septations and calcifications may be present.

✓ **Pearls and ✗ Pitfalls**

✓ Magnetic resonance imaging is better than other modalities at showing cyst complexity.
✓ Nodular enhancement or thick septations would suggest malignancy.
✗ Biliary hamartomas can occur in men (female:male ratio of 9:1).
✗ The lesion may mimic an abscess.

Case 19

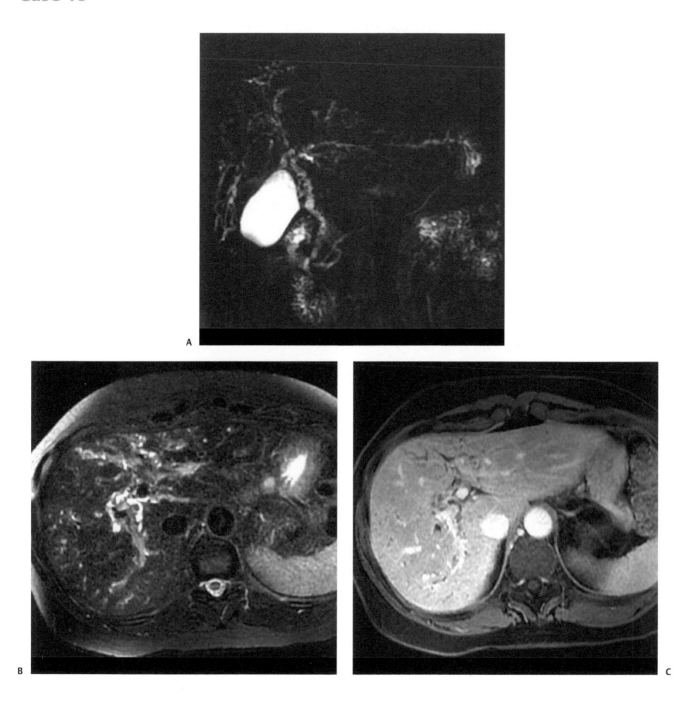

■ Clinical Presentation

A 70-year-old female with elevated liver function tests.

■ **Imaging Findings**

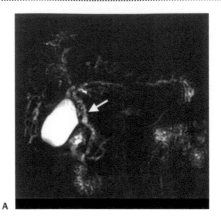 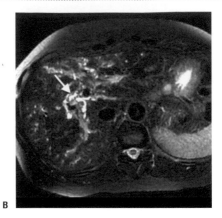 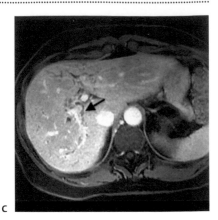

A   B   C

(A) Coronal magnetic resonance cholangiopancreatography (MRCP) shows multiple strictures in the intrahepatic and extrahepatic biliary tree (*arrow*). **(B)** Axial T2 fat-saturated image shows areas of intrahepatic biliary ductal dilation (*arrow*). **(C)** Axial T1-fast spoiled gradient echo with contrast shows enhancement of the bile duct walls (*arrow*).

■ **Differential Diagnosis**

• ***Primary sclerosing cholangitis (PSC):*** Chronic liver disease characterized by inflammation and fibrosis of the intra- and extrahepatic biliary tree resulting in cholestasis and increased risk for cholangiocarcinoma.
• *Primary biliary cholangitis:* Rare autoimmune disease of the liver. It occurs primarily in females and where there is chronic progressive destruction of the small intrahepatic bile ducts. This leads to cholestasis and hepatic fibrosis. There are usually no changes in the biliary tree on imaging studies.

■ **Essential Facts**

• PSC is an autoimmune disease that causes inflammation and fibrosis of the intra- and extrahepatic biliary tree resulting in chronic cholestasis.
• The primary concern in imaging these patients is the development of cholangiocarcinoma with a prevalence of 7–13%.
• Patients must undergo periodic screening to evaluate for the development of malignancy or dominant strictures. A new or developing mass, dominant stricture, or asymmetric ductal dilation requires further evaluation with endoscopic retrograde cholangiopancreatography (ERCP).

• PSC can be seen in the setting of inflammatory bowel disease (IBD), and ~75 to 95% of patients with PSC have IBD.
• Hepatic transplant is performed in some cases with relapse rates of ~15%.

■ **Other Imaging Findings**

• Ultrasound may detect scattered biliary dilation, or the imaging findings may mimic cirrhosis.
• On computed tomography, small scattered dilated ducts or a focal mass may be detected.
• MRCP is the imaging modality of choice to evaluate the biliary tree.

✓ **Pearls and ✗ Pitfalls**

✓ Magnetic resonance imaging/MRCP is the modality of choice to noninvasively image the biliary tree.
✓ New or dominant strictures should be further worked up with ERCP and can be found in 20% of cases.
✗ Small masses can cause malignant stricturing.
✗ Enhancement and thickening of the biliary tree wall can be seen in cholangitis.

Case 20

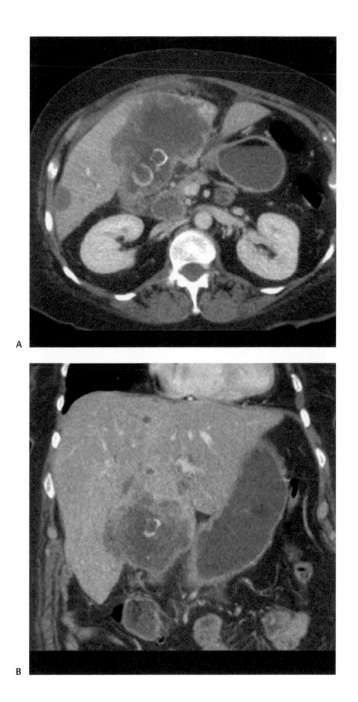

A

B

▪ Clinical Presentation

A 75-year-old female with right upper quadrant pain and weight loss.

■ **Imaging Findings**

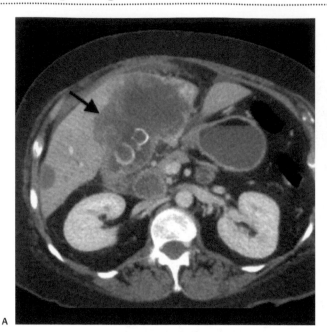 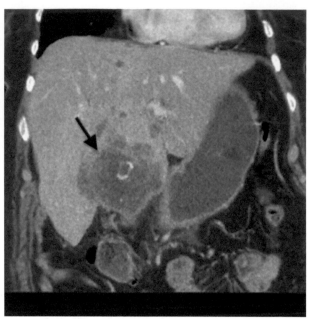

(A) Axial contrast-enhanced computed tomography (CT) shows stones in the gallbladder with a fundal mass that invades the liver (*arrow*). **(B)** Coronal contrast-enhanced CT shows multiple hypodense lesions in the liver in addition to the dominant mass in the gallbladder fossa (*arrow*).

■ **Differential Diagnosis**

- ***Gallbladder carcinoma:*** A malignant neoplasm that arises from the gallbladder wall that tends to spread early to lymph nodes and liver and has a poor prognosis unless detected early.
- *Cholangiocarcinoma with gallbladder invasion:* Secondary invasion of the gallbladder occurs when hepatic lesions cross the capsule and enter the wall and lumen of the gallbladder.

■ **Essential Facts**

- Gallbladder carcinoma is most commonly caused by adenocarcinoma of the gallbladder (90%); the remainder of the lesions are squamous cell carcinoma.
- Gallbladder carcinoma is the most common malignancy of the biliary tree after cholangiocarcinoma.
- The most common risk factors include chronic cholecystitis, cholelithiasis (present in about 85% of patients), chronic inflammation, and porcelain gallbladder with calcification involving the mucosa.
- Patients with biliary inflammation such as primary sclerosing cholangitis and inflammatory bowel disease are at increased risk of malignancy.
- Prognosis is poor as the mass tends to invade the liver and hepatic hilar nodes early. Hepatic metastatic disease has a dismal prognosis.

■ **Other Imaging Findings**

- Ultrasound may show a polypoid mass or a mass that fills the lumen of the gallbladder, but porcelain gallbladder or cholelithiasis can obscure the evaluation of the gallbladder due to shadowing. Magnetic resonance imaging/magnetic resonance cholangiopancreatography is an excellent modality to image the gallbladder and biliary tree. The use of subtraction imaging can help detect mural enhancement. F18–fluorodeoxyglucose positron emission tomography/CT is useful in the staging of gallbladder carcinoma as the primary lesion; metastatic deposits are FDG avid.

✓ **Pearls and ✗ Pitfalls**

- ✓ Gallbladder carcinoma can present as a mass that replaces the lumen of the gallbladder.
- ✓ Gallbladder carcinoma can present as a polypoid mass or asymmetric wall thickening.
- ✗ It is important not to mistake cholecystitis for gallbladder carcinoma.
- ✗ Peritoneal and omental metastases can be missed on preoperative imaging.

Case 21

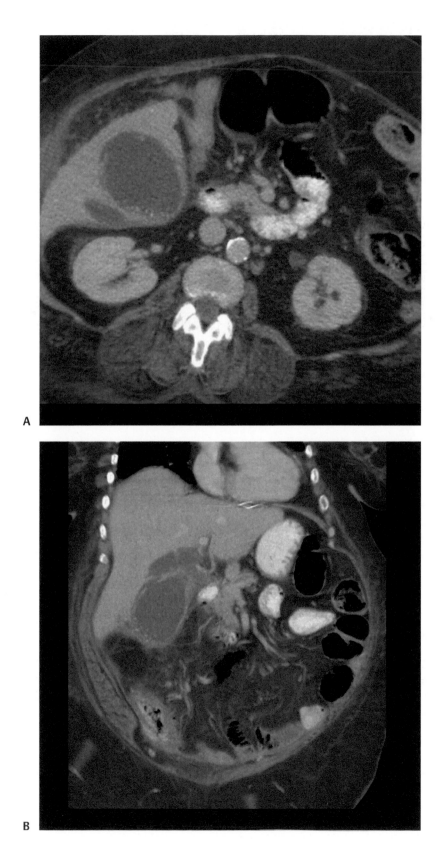

A

B

A 72-year-old female with abdominal pain.

■ Imaging Findings

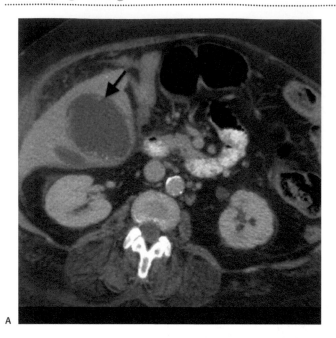
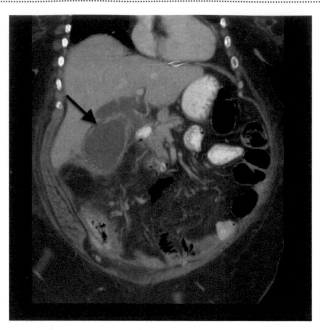

A　　　　　　　　　　　　　　　　　　　　　　　　　　　　　　　　　　　　B

Axial **(A)** and coronal **(B)** contrast-enhanced computed tomography (CT) of the abdomen shows a distended gallbladder with stones, discontinuous wall, intraluminal membranes, pericholecystic fluid, and a small fluid collection near the liver (*arrows*).

■ Differential Diagnosis

- ***Gangrenous cholecystitis:*** Acute severe transmural inflammation and ischemic necrosis of the gallbladder wall that can lead to rupture and abscess formation. This is a complication of acute cholecystitis.
- *Acute cholecystitis:* Acute inflammation of the gallbladder. It is commonly caused by cholelithiasis and obstruction of the cystic duct.

■ Essential Facts

- Gangrenous cholecystitis is more common in older males with cardiovascular disease and diabetes.
- The gallbladder is frequently distended and shows areas of poor wall enhancement.
- The imaging findings most associated with gangrenous cholecystitis are gas in the wall or lumen, intraluminal membranes, irregular or absent wall, and abscess.
- Contrast-enhanced CT detects gangrenous cholecystitis with a reported accuracy of 87%.

■ Other Imaging Findings

- Ultrasound is superior to CT for identifying stones in the gallbladder.
- In cases of gangrenous cholecystitis, gas in the wall is detected as echogenic layers with posterior "dirty shadow."
- A thick striated wall, lack of color flow in the wall, and surrounding fluid collections are other ultrasound imaging findings. Technetium^{99m} di-isoimmino-diacetic acid can be falsely negative in cases of gangrenous cholecystitis.

✓ Pearls and ✗ Pitfalls

- ✓ Use coronal and axial images to ensure the gallbladder wall is intact.
- ✓ Look for early abscess formation and signs of perforation.
- ✗ Noncontrast CT may miss important findings.
- ✗ Stones may not be evident on CT.

Case 22

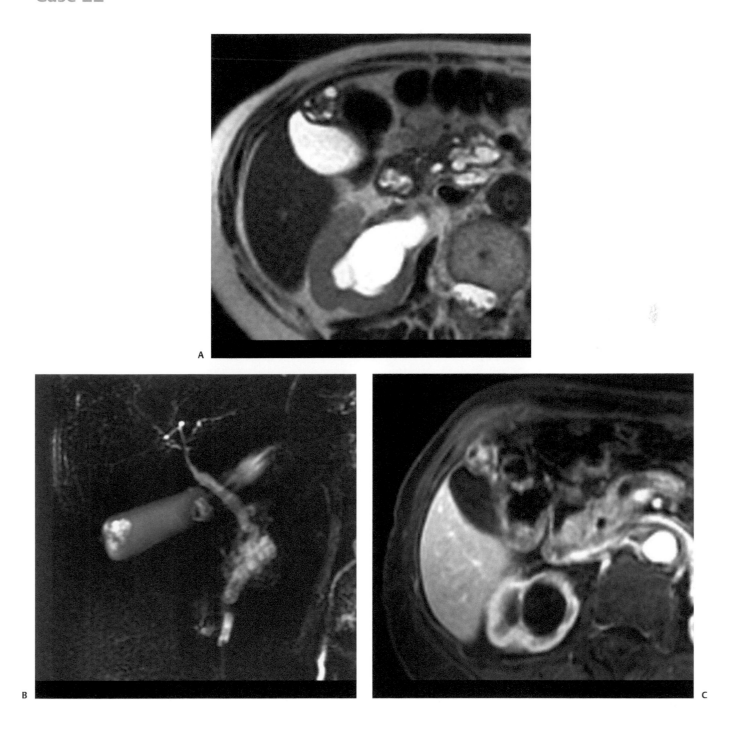

A

B

C

■ Clinical Presentation

A 75-year-old female with an incidentally detected gallbladder mass.

■ **Imaging Findings**

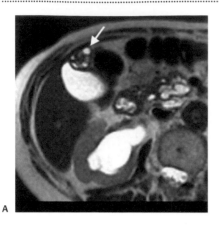 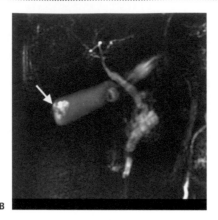 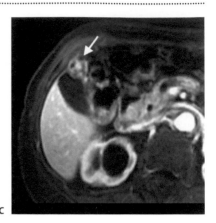

A   B   C

(A) Axial T2-weighted image of the gallbladder shows a focal fundal mass that has several T2-hyperintense cystic spaces (*arrow*). **(B)** Coronal magnetic resonance cholangiopancreatography shows the multicystic mass at the fundus of the gallbladder (*arrow*). **(C)** Contrast-enhanced axial T1-fast spoiled gradient echo shows wall enhancement and central nodular enhancement in the lesion (*arrow*).

■ **Differential Diagnosis**

- ***Adenomyomatosis of the gallbladder:*** A benign entity of the gallbladder wall formed by excessive epithelial proliferation and hyperplasia of the muscularis propria. This leads to epithelial in-folding within the muscular layer resulting in diverticular pouches called Rokitansky-Aschoff sinuses that are lined with epithelium.
- *Gallbladder carcinoma:* A malignant neoplasm that arises from the gallbladder wall that tends to spread to lymph nodes and liver early and has a poor prognosis unless detected early.

■ **Essential Facts**

- Adenomyomatosis comprises dilated diverticular pouches lined with epithelium, producing a characteristic "cystic" appearance.
- The distribution can be one of four types. Localized (as in this case) occurs at the fundus and is the most common. Annular occurs in the mid-gallbladder as a ring causing a waist in the gallbladder shape. Segmental affects a segment of the gallbladder wall, typically the fundus and a third of the wall. Diffuse affects the entire wall, and the gallbladder has a contracted appearance.
- Bile deposition can lead to bile crystal deposition that can calcify in the wall over time, producing the classic "comet tail" artifact on ultrasound.

■ **Other Imaging Findings**

- Ultrasound can show the cystic spaces or the reverberation artifact that produces the typical "comet tail" artifact and helps confirm the diagnosis. Computed tomography (CT) may depict the cystic spaces in the wall. However, when these are absent, adenomyomatosis is difficult to differentiate from early gallbladder carcinoma.

✓ **Pearls and ✗ Pitfalls**

- ✓ The key to diagnosis is the identification of the cystic spaces on magnetic resonance imaging (MRI) with an appearance referred to as a "pearl necklace" or on CT with an appearance referred to as a "rosary."
- ✓ It is seen in older patients, typically females.
- ✗ Early gallbladder carcinoma can present as a fundal mass but lacks the typical cystic spaces.
- ✗ Lesions that are new, change in a short period, or show signs of aggressive behavior must be considered malignant.

Case 23

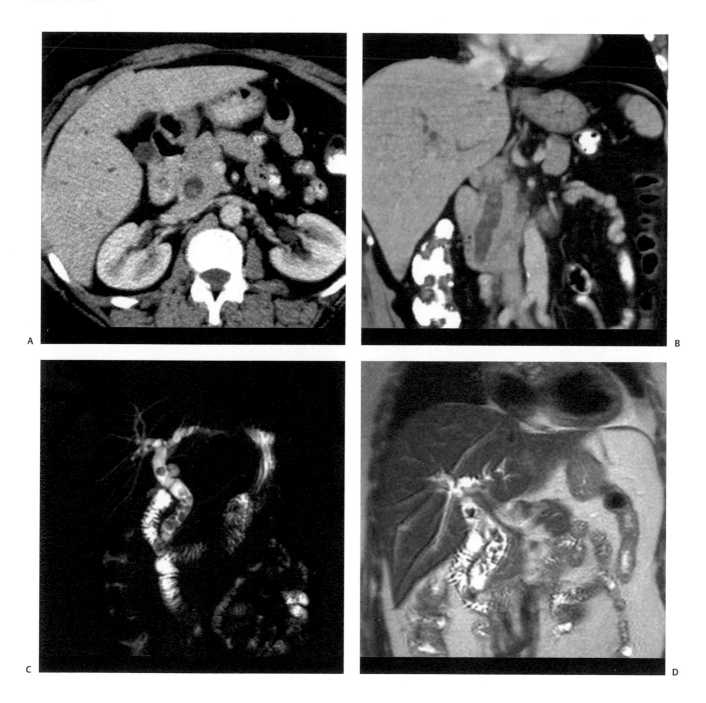

■ Clinical Presentation

A 54-year-old female with history of cholecystectomy and right upper quadrant pain.

■ **Imaging Findings**

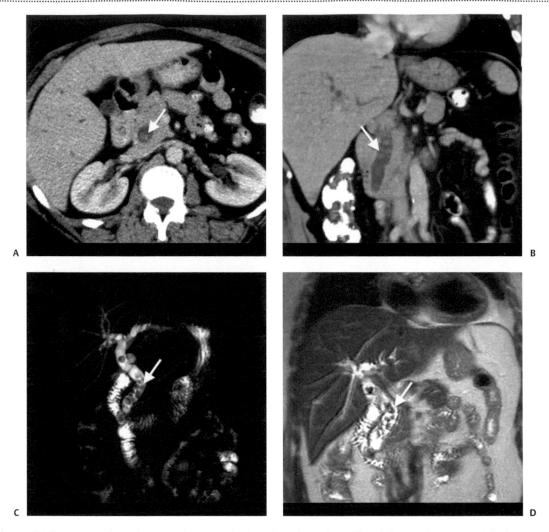

A   B   C   D

Axial **(A)** and coronal **(B)** contrast-enhanced computed tomography (CT) shows hyperdense filling defects in the common bile duct (CBD) to the level of the ampulla (*arrows*). Note the crescent appearance of bile around the stone. **(C)** Coronal T2 magnetic resonance cholangiopancreatography (MRCP) shows multiple filling defects in the CBD (*arrow*). **(D)** Coronal T2 single shot fast spin echo shows the biliary stones as dark filling defects (*arrow*).

■ **Differential Diagnosis**

• **Choledocholithiasis:** Biliary stones in the CBD that can cause biliary obstruction or infection.

■ **Essential Facts**

• Choledocholithiasis is present in 6 to 12% of cases undergoing cholecystectomy.
• Recurrent choledocholithiasis occurs in 14% of patients after stone removal and drainage by endoscopic retrograde cholangiopancreatography.
• Choledocholithiasis can cause biliary obstruction, biliary infection, and pancreatitis. It can occur following cholecystectomy and would require biliary imaging.
• MRCP is excellent at detecting choledocholithiasis; stones are identified as dark filling defects on T2-weighed imaging.

■ **Other Imaging Findings**

• Ultrasound can detect choledocholithiasis as filling defects in the CBD. However, the entirety of the CBD may not be imaged due to bowel gas.

✓ **Pearls and** ✗ **Pitfalls**

✓ Use coronal images to view the CBD along its length to evaluate for choledocholithiasis.
✓ Proper window and level settings are needed to evaluate choledocholithiasis.
✗ Small stones near the ampulla can be missed on CT, magnetic resonance imaging, or ultrasound.
✗ Noncalcified stones can be difficult to identify on CT.

Case 24

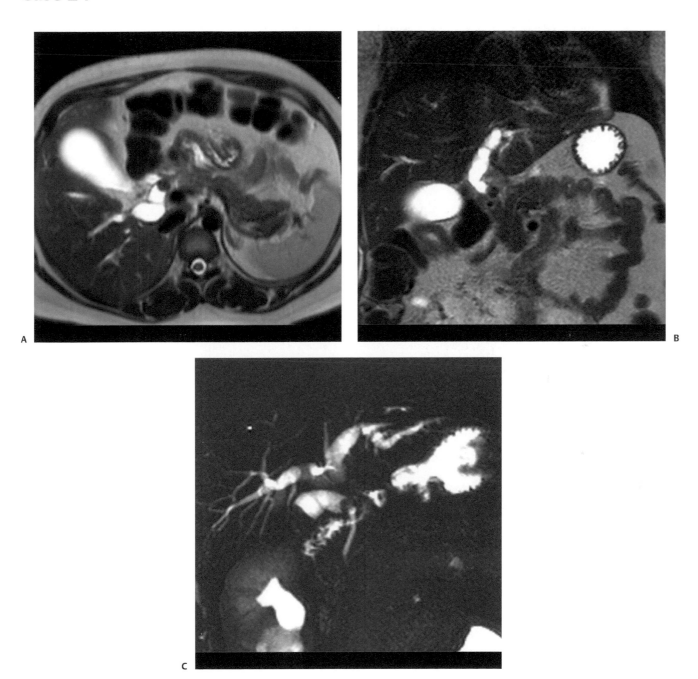

A

B

C

■ Clinical Presentation

A 24-year-old female with right upper quadrant pain and jaundice.

■ Imaging Findings

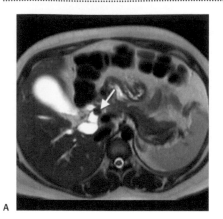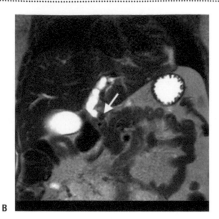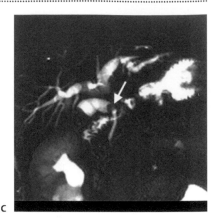

A   B   C

(A) Axial T2-weighted single shot fast spin echo (SSFSE) shows a filling defect in a dilated cystic duct (*arrow*). **(B)** Coronal T2-weighted SSFSE shows the filling defect in the cystic duct as well as intrahepatic ductal dilation (*arrow*). **(C)** Coronal T2-weighted magnetic resonance cholangiopancreatography (MRCP) shows the stone in the cystic duct as the site of obstruction with intrahepatic ductal dilation proximally and normal appearing common bile duct distally (*arrow*).

■ Differential Diagnosis

- **Mirizzi's syndrome:** Obstructive jaundice due to an impacted stone either in the cystic duct or the neck of the gallbladder that causes intrahepatic biliary ductal dilation.
- *Choledocholithiasis:* Biliary calculi in the common bile duct.

■ Essential Facts

- Mirizzi's syndrome is a complication of gallstone disease.
- The obstructing stone is in the gallbladder neck or the cystic duct and causes extrinsic compression of the common duct.
- The gallbladder and intrahepatic ducts are dilated in the setting of cholelithiasis.
- There is inflammation of the triangle of Calot (bounded by the hepatic surface, common hepatic duct, and cystic duct).
- Complications include formation of biliary-enteric fistulae and an increased risk of gallbladder malignancy.

■ Other Imaging Findings

- Ultrasound can identify the stone lodged in the cystic duct and the intrahepatic ductal dilation.
- On ultrasound, the common bile duct near the head of the pancreas is normal in caliber.
- Ultrasound may not identify complications such as fistulae.

✓ Pearls and ✗ Pitfalls

✓ MRCP is an excellent modality to detect the biliary obstruction and stone(s) associated with Mirizzi's syndrome.

✓ Mirizzi's syndrome can be associated with cholecystitis.

✗ Inflammation of the gallbladder or the cystic duct can masquerade as malignancy.

✗ Endoscopic retrograde cholangiopancreatography may not identify the stone because it is not in the common bile duct and instead is found in the cystic duct or gallbladder neck.

Case 25

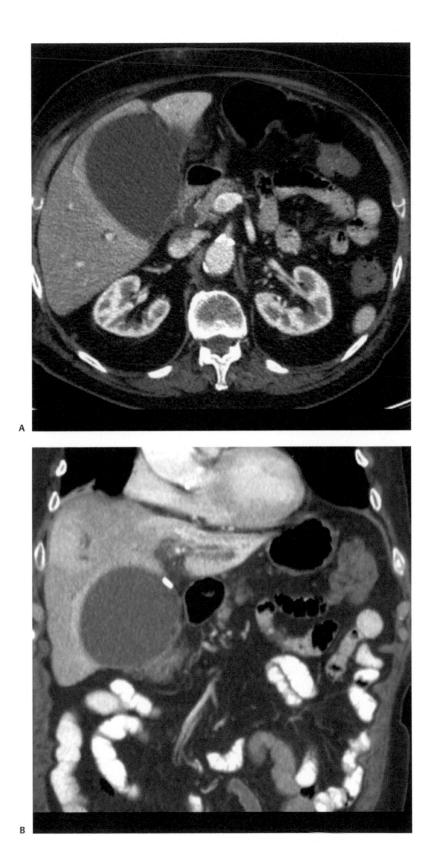

A

B

■ Clinical Presentation

An 84-year-old patient with fever and abdominal pain after cholecystectomy.

■ Imaging Findings

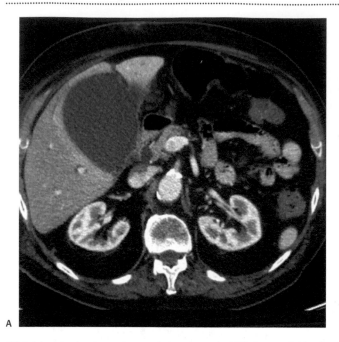

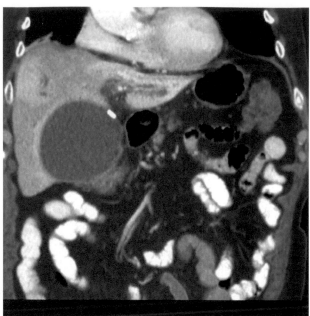

(A) Axial contrast-enhanced computed tomography (CT) shows a fluid collection in the gallbladder fossa. **(B)** Coronal contrast-enhanced CT shows a fluid collection in the gallbladder fossa. There are areas of hyperenhancement in the hepatic parenchyma.

■ Differential Diagnosis

- **Biloma:** Collections of bile that are found outside the biliary tree. They can be located inside or outside of the liver.
- *Abscess:* Collection of infected, suppurative material usually with a wall.

■ Essential Facts

- Bilomas are most commonly secondary to biliary injury during cholecystectomy and occur in ~7% of cases.
- Other causes include radiofrequency ablation, chemoembolization, liver resection, biliary anastomotic leak, and trauma.
- On CT, bilomas are near fluid attenuating with an average density of 20 Hounsfield units. They can be focal collections in the gallbladder fossa or around the liver surface, or they can be diffuse within the abdomen.
- They are treated with percutaneous drainage if the collection is large or the patient is symptomatic.
- Bilomas can form days to weeks after the initial biliary injury.

■ Other Imaging Findings

- Ultrasound can depict fluid collections in and around the liver. It can be used as a modality to guide percutaneous drainage of the collection.
- Hepatobiliary cholescintigraphy is useful to detect or confirm a biloma but poor at delineating biliary anatomy.

- Accumulation of radiotracer confirms biloma, but 4-hour and 24-hour imaging may be needed to detect slow leaks. Magnetic resonance cholangiopancreatography is excellent for the detection of collections in and around the liver. The signal intensity of the collection may help distinguish between fluid collections such as abscess, pseudocyst, biloma, or hematoma. Bilomas can show concentrated layering (bile has high signal on T1 and low signal on T2).
- Endoscopic retrograde cholangiopancreatography (ERCP) can confirm extravasation of contrast into the collection and help define the anatomy.

✓ Pearls and ✗ Pitfalls

- ✓ CT scan with contrast is excellent for the detection of bilomas.
- ✓ Fluid collections in the liver that are new and near the biliary tree may represent intrahepatic bilomas in patients who have undergone biliary or hepatic intervention.
- ✗ CT scan may not be able to differentiate between evolving hematoma, abscess, and bilomas.
- ✗ Fluid collections in the gallbladder fossa may mimic a native gallbladder; proper history is important.

Case 26

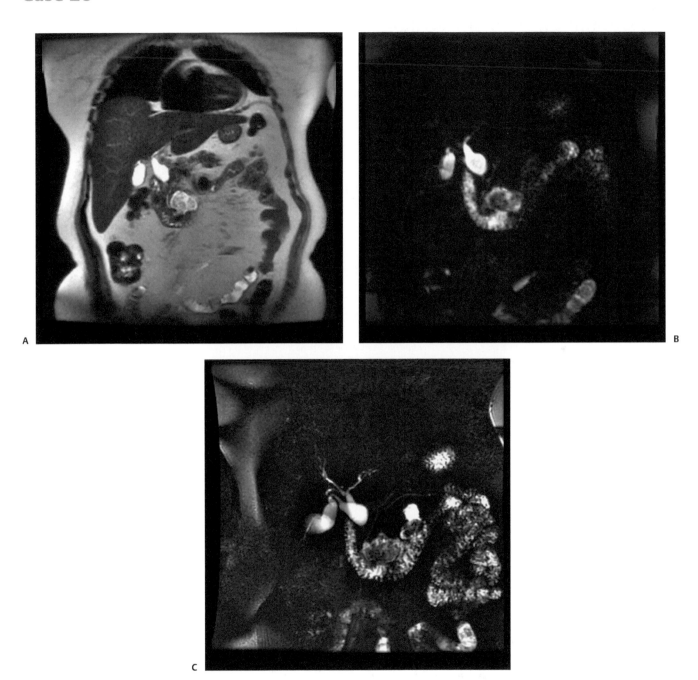

A

B

C

■ Clinical Presentation

An elderly female with biliary abnormality undergoes magnetic resonance imaging (MRI)/magnetic resonance cholangio-pancreatography (MRCP).

■ **Imaging Findings**

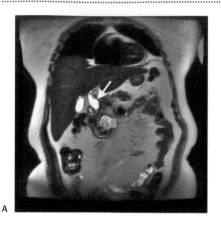 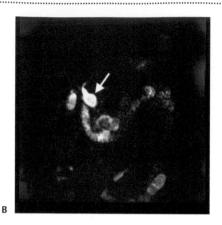 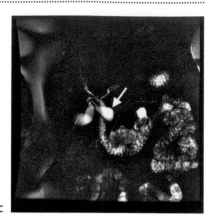

A   B   C

(A) Coronal single shot fast spin echo T2 shows a fusiform dilated common bile duct (CBD) and no intrahepatic ductal dilation (*arrow*). **(B)** Coronal thin-slice MRCP shows the ductal dilation of the common hepatic duct (*arrow*). **(C)** Coronal MRCP shows the fusiform dilation of the CBD, involving the common hepatic duct (*arrow*).

■ **Differential Diagnosis**

- ***Choledochal cyst type I:*** Congenital abnormality associated with anomalous union of the pancreatic and biliary ducts and evidenced by dilation of the extrahepatic bile ducts.
- *Biliary obstruction:* Biliary obstruction results in dilation of the biliary tree proximal to a site of obstruction.

■ **Essential Facts**

- Choledochal cysts are caused by anomalous union of the pancreatic and biliary ducts outside the duodenal wall and proximal to the sphincter of Oddi, resulting in reflux into the biliary tree.
- Choledochal cysts are more common in females (4:1).
- The Todani classification separates choledochal cysts into five main types.
- Biliary malignancy is the major risk factor in these cases, and screening is indicated.
- Other risk factors include cholecystitis, recurrent cholangitis, biliary stricture, choledocholithiasis, and recurrent acute pancreatitis.
- Types I and IV are most associated with malignancy. Type V is also known as Caroli's disease.

■ **Other Imaging Findings**

- Ultrasound can detect CBD dilation.
- Intrahepatic ductal dilation may be mistaken for a cyst if focal.
- Endoscopic retrograde cholangiopancreatography is the gold standard for evaluation of the biliary tree.

✓ **Pearls and** ✗ **Pitfalls**

- ✓ Thin-section and thick-section MRCP images should be used to evaluate the biliary tree.
- ✓ Screening using MRI is needed to detect malignancy.
- ✗ Biliary stones can be mistaken for malignancy; postcontrast imaging should be used.
- ✗ The shape of the CBD should be evaluated and not mistaken for the chronic biliary dilation that can be seen in the elderly or after cholecystectomy.

Case 27

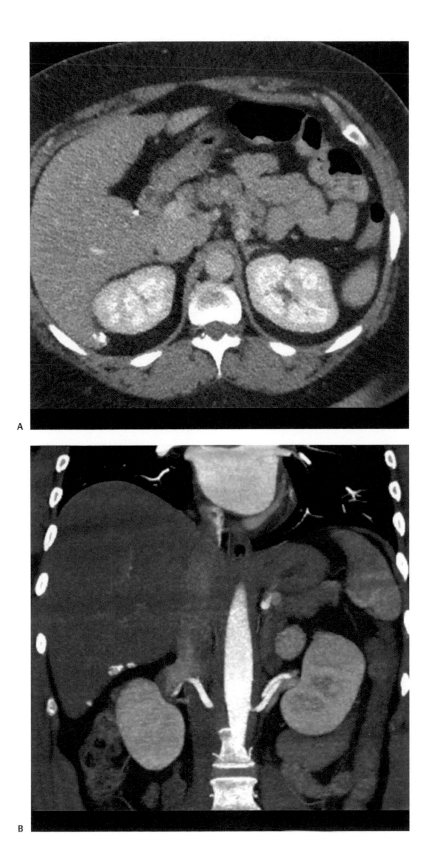

■ Clinical Presentation

A 51-year-old female with right upper quadrant pain. Patient has a history of laparoscopic cholecystectomy.

■ **Imaging Findings**

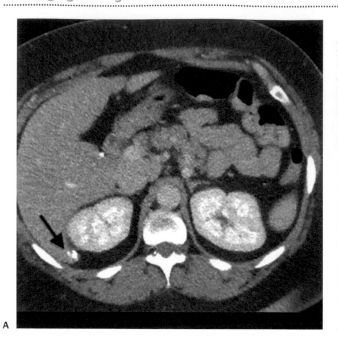
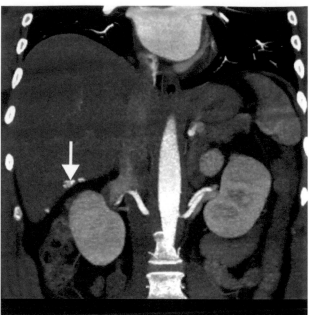

(A) Axial contrast-enhanced computed tomography (CT) shows an empty gallbladder fossa and a calcification in the fossa and Morrison's pouch (*arrow*). **(B)** Coronal maximum intensity projection CT shows multiple stones near the right hepatic margin (*arrow*).

■ **Differential Diagnosis**

• ***Dropped gallstones:*** Dropped gallstones can result from a spillage of gallbladder contents into the abdomen from laparoscopic cholecystectomy.

■ **Essential Facts**

• Dropped gallstones can occur following spillage of gallbladder contents.
• The stones are seen in the gallbladder fossa, Morrison's pouch, and the pelvis.
• Although most are silent and incidentally detected, they can cause pain from inflammation or infection and, in some cases, abscess.

■ **Other Imaging Findings**

• Ultrasound may detect these stones near the liver as echogenic foci with posterior shadowing.
• On magnetic resonance imaging, the stones are usually hypointense because they are calcified; they may be associated with surrounding soft tissue enhancement.

✓ **Pearls and ✗ Pitfalls**

✓ Calcifications outside the gallbladder and near the liver that resemble stones can represent dropped gallstones.
✓ The cause may not always be surgical and can also be seen in the setting of gallbladder perforation.
✗ The stones can be associated with inflammatory soft tissue and should not be confused with peritoneal deposits.
✗ Rarely, they can be located in the body wall and can form a fistula.

Case 28

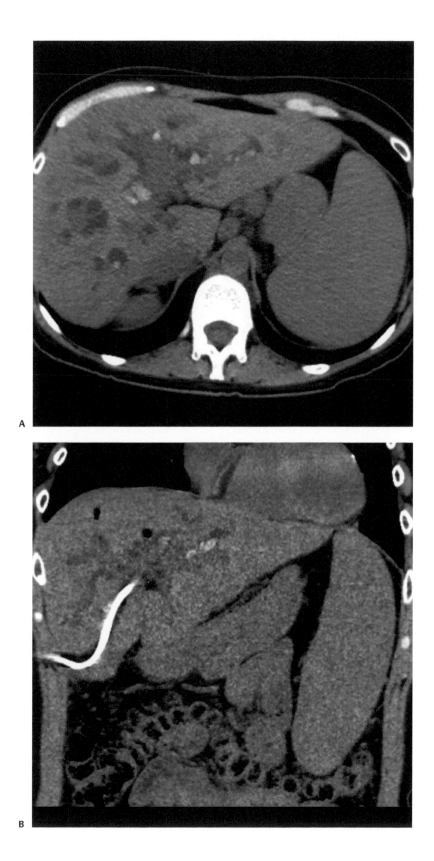

■ Clinical Presentation

A 50-year-old female with recurrent bouts of fever and cholangitis.

■ Imaging Findings

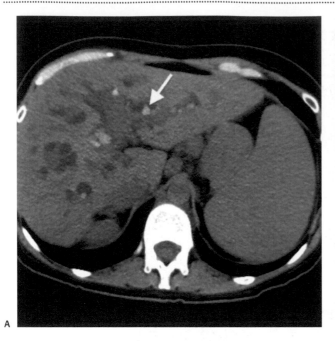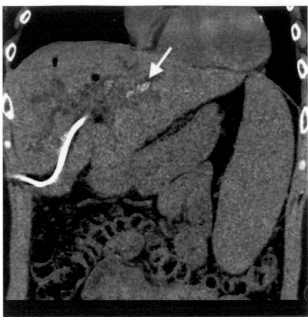

A   B

(A) Axial computed tomography (CT) shows radiodense stones in the dilated biliary tree (*arrow*). **(B)** Coronal CT shows radiodense stones and a biliary drainage catheter to decompress the biliary tree (*arrow*).

■ Differential Diagnosis

- **Hepatolithiasis:** Biliary stones in the intrahepatic bile ducts.
- *Biliary hemorrhage:* Hemorrhagic products in the biliary tree.
- *Caroli disease:* Congenital focal dilation of the biliary tree, which can have biliary lithiasis.

■ Essential Facts

- Hepatolithiasis is endemic to East Asia with a prevalence ranging as high as 30–50%.
- The etiology is multifactorial, including genetic, dietary, and environmental factors.
- It causes recurrent cholangitis, biliary strictures, liver abscesses, and atrophy or cirrhosis of the affected liver.
- Hepatolithiasis is associated with an increased risk of cholangiocarcinoma.
- Type 1 is localized stone disease, either unilobar or bilobar; type 2 is diffuse stone disease.
- The stones are brown pigment stones as well as cholesterol stones.

■ Other Imaging Findings

- Magnetic resonance cholangiopancreatography is excellent at depicting the biliary tree and the filling defects. Both radiopaque and nonradiopaque stones can be imaged. The ultrasound shows the intrahepatic stones as shadowing foci with associated ductal dilation.

✓ Pearls and ✗ Pitfalls

- ✓ Noncontrast CT is useful in locating the stones in the biliary tree.
- ✓ Knowledge of biliary anatomy and accurate description of stone burden will help therapy.
- ✗ Patients with new strictures or new biliary ductal dilation should be scrutinized for malignancy.
- ✗ Biliary enhancement may be present in the setting of cholangitis and should not be mistaken for malignancy.

Case 29

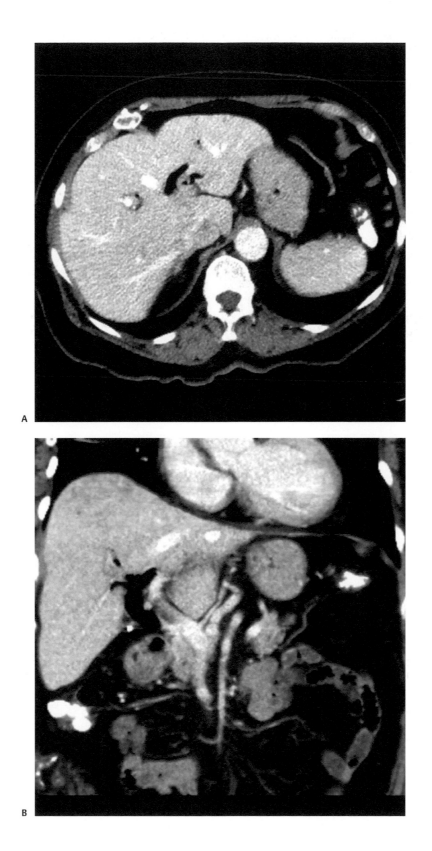

A

B

■ Clinical Presentation

An 82-year-old female with fever and right upper quadrant pain after endoscopic retrograde cholangiopancreatography (ERCP).

■ **Imaging Findings**

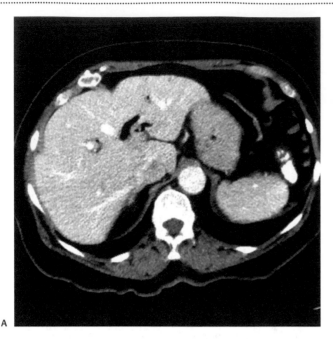
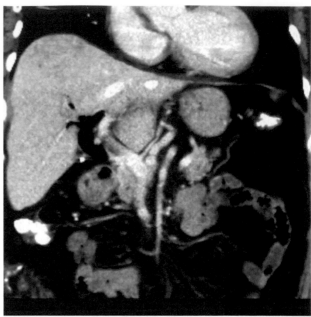

(A) Axial contrast-enhanced computed tomography (CT) shows expected pneumobilia and patent vessels. **(B)** Coronal contrast-enhanced CT shows perfusional changes along the periphery of the liver.

■ **Differential Diagnosis**

- **Cholangitis:** Acute bacterial infection of the biliary tract that can be caused by biliary obstruction, malignancy, or biliary procedures.
- *Hepatic abscess:* Areas of infected liver that have undergone necrosis. CT demonstrates multiple, low-level attenuating lesions with wall enhancement and perfusion abnormality.

■ **Essential Facts**

- The classic presentation is fever, jaundice, and right upper quadrant pain.
- The causes are choledocholithiasis, malignancy, immunocompromise, and bacteria introduced via biliary procedures.
- Most infections are polymicrobial with gram-negative rods found in up to 88%.
- Development of cholangitis requires bacterial contamination of the bile ducts, stagnant bile, and increased intrabiliary pressure.
- Imaging features include biliary wall enhancement, wall thickening, and ductal obstruction.
- Heterogeneous perfusion can be seen in the liver parenchyma distal to the infected ducts. In immunocompromised patients, cholangitis can be caused by human immunodeficiency virus and other atypical infectious agents.

- Subacute cholangitis can be seen in the setting of liver transplant.
- The primary complications are sepsis, hepatic abscesses, portal vein thrombosis, and bile peritonitis.
- Chronic bacterial cholangitis can result in portal vein thrombosis, biliary stricture, sclerosing cholangitis, and cholangiocarcinoma.

■ **Other Imaging Findings**

- Ultrasound can show dilated ducts or abscess formation.
- Magnetic resonance imaging with contrast is an excellent tool for elevating the biliary tree for enhancement and thickening associated with cholangitis.

✓ **Pearls and** ✗ **Pitfalls**

- ✓ Contrast-enhanced CT is recommended for diagnosis.
- ✓ Use of coronal images is helpful in evaluating the biliary tree.
- ✗ Early liver abscess formation and advanced cholangitis may have a similar appearance.
- ✗ Portal vein thrombosis and hepatic abscess can be silent and may only be discovered at imaging.

Case 30

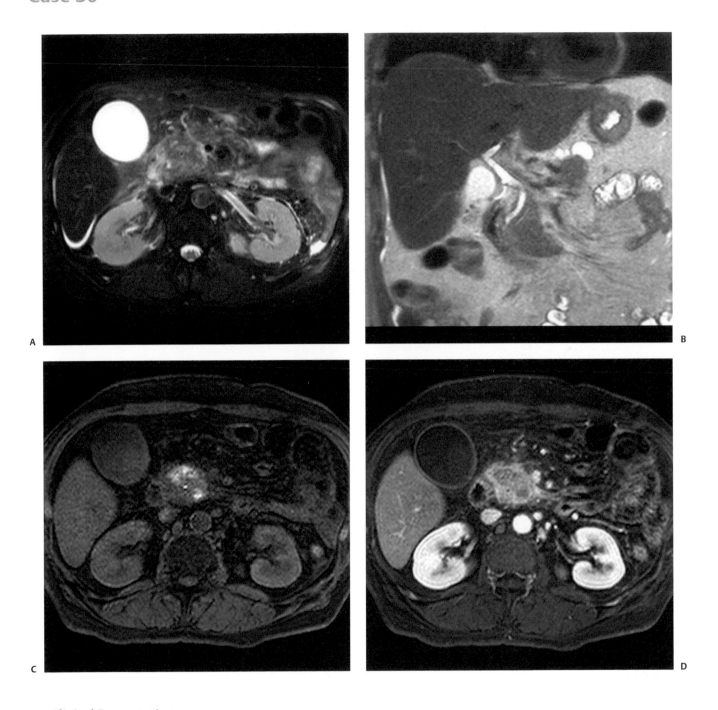

A

B

C

D

■ Clinical Presentation

A 54-year-old male with abdominal pain and elevated amylase and lipase.

■ Imaging Findings

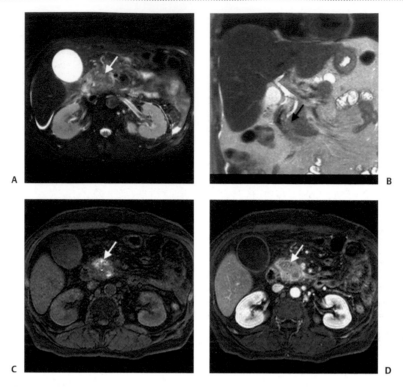

(A) Axial T2 fat-saturated image shows edema in the head of the pancreas and upper abdominal ascites (*arrow*). **(B)** Coronal T2 shows edema in the head of the pancreas and no ductal dilation (*arrow*). **(C)** Axial T1-fast spoiled gradient echo (FSPGR) shows two patchy areas of T1 hyperintensity in the edematous pancreatic head (*arrow*). **(D)** Axial T1-FSPGR + contrast shows decreased enhancement in the head corresponding to the areas of T1 hyperintensity (*arrow*).

■ Differential Diagnosis

• ***Acute pancreatitis with necrosis:*** Acute pancreatitis is acute inflammation of the pancreas resulting in acinar cell injury and activation of pancreatic enzymes.

■ Essential Facts

• Acute pancreatitis is characterized by pancreatic inflammation and acinar cell injury that leads to activation of pancreatic enzymes. Pancreatic necrosis is a complication in ~20–30% of cases.
• Acute pancreatitis has increased T2 signal that is best imaged on the fat-saturated T2-weighted images.
• There is loss of the normal high-T1 intrinsic acinar protein signal in acute pancreatitis.
• Parenchymal hemorrhage is seen as the spotted or patchy areas of hyperintensity on T1-weighted images with fat suppression. A hypointense hemosiderin rim is typically seen on T2-weighted images.

■ Other Imaging Findings

• Computed tomography (CT) with contrast is excellent at identifying acute pancreatitis and its associated complications.

• Findings include fluid in the surrounding tissues and edematous parenchyma.
• Gas in a collection suggestive of abscess is better seen on CT.
• Ultrasound may detect pancreatic edema by a loss of hyperechogenicity that is seen in the pancreas or peripancreatic fluid.

✓ Pearls and ✗ Pitfalls

✓ The most sensitive sequence for identifying fluid collections is T2-weighted fat-suppressed images.
✓ Precontrast T1-FSPGR images with patchy areas of hyperintensity can be used to identify hemorrhage.
✗ Pancreatic necrosis may be difficult to diagnose as the pancreas is intrinsically T1-hyperintense and can be mistaken for enhancing tissue.
✗ Focal mass-like enlargement of the pancreas in the setting of acute inflammation should not be mistaken for malignancy. Follow-up imaging after the acute pancreatitis has resolved will determine if there is an underlying malignancy in cases where the etiology is undetermined.

Case 31

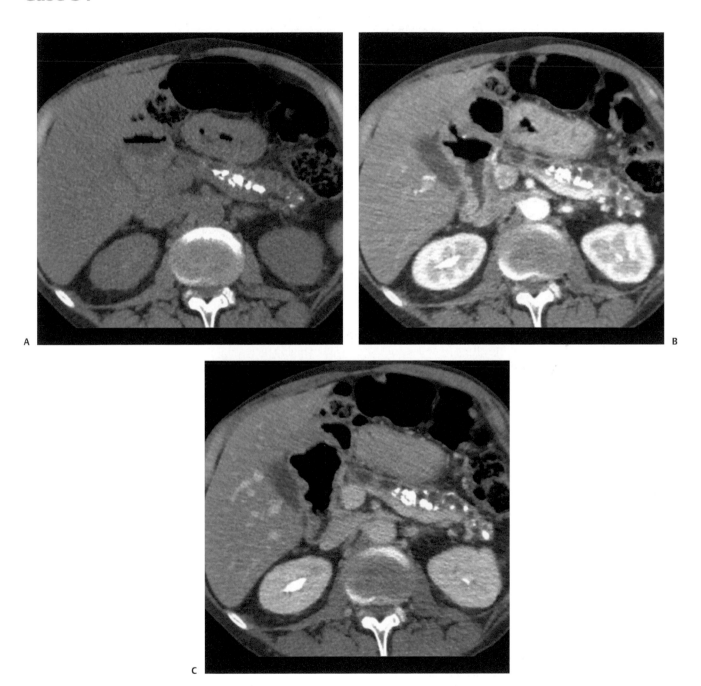

A

B

C

■ Clinical Presentation

A 60-year-old male with chronic abdominal pain and weight loss.

■ **Imaging Findings**

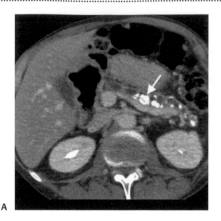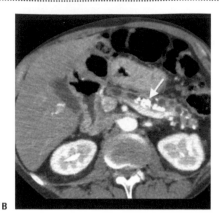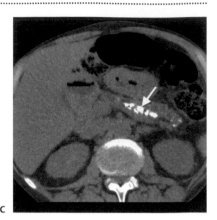

(A) Noncontrast computed tomography (CT) shows multiple stones in the pancreatic duct and parenchyma (*arrow*). **(B)** Contrast-enhanced CT shows advanced pancreatic atrophy, a dilated main duct, and poor pancreatic parenchymal enhancement (*arrow*). **(C)** Delayed phase CT shows enhancement of the parenchyma, which can be seen in fibrosis (*arrow*).

■ **Differential Diagnosis**

• ***Chronic pancreatitis:*** A progressive inflammatory process involving the pancreas, resulting in endocrine and exocrine gland dysfunction and fibrosis.

■ **Essential Facts**

• Chronic pancreatitis occurs as a result of chronic inflammation of the gland. It can be idiopathic, but risk factors include alcohol abuse, genetic predisposition, and stone disease.
• CT findings include gland atrophy and fibrosis.
• The main pancreatic duct is usually dilated and irregular. The dilation can be segmental or entire.
• Calcified stones occur in the body and main duct. Coexisting stones in the parenchyma and duct make the diagnosis for chronic pancreatitis definite.
• Complications include chronic pancreatic pseudocysts, poor endocrine and exocrine function, and splenic vein and mesenteric vein thrombosis.

■ **Other Imaging Findings**

• Magnetic resonance imaging (MRI)/magnetic resonance cholangiopancreatography (MRCP) will show a dilated duct and stones as filling defects. There can be restricted diffusion in the parenchyma due to fibrosis.
• Ultrasound shows an echogenic gland with the stones as echogenic foci with posterior acoustic shadowing.

✓ **Pearls and ✗ Pitfalls**

✓ A pancreatic mass should be excluded.
✓ Secretin MRCP is useful in evaluating the exocrine capacity of the gland.
✗ The dilated duct should not be confused with a main branch type intraductal papillary or mucinous tumor.
✗ Calcifications in the duct and parenchyma may not be identified on MRI.

Case 32

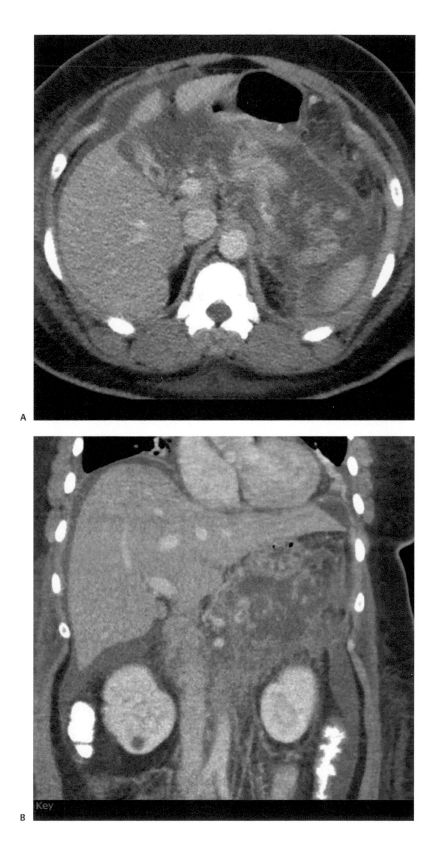

■ Clinical Presentation

A 51-year-old female with acute abdominal pain.

■ **Imaging Findings**

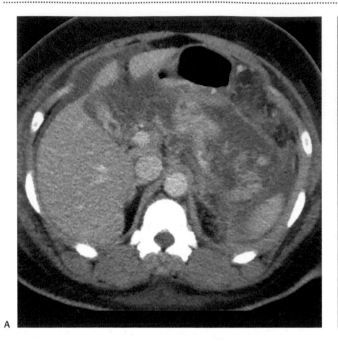 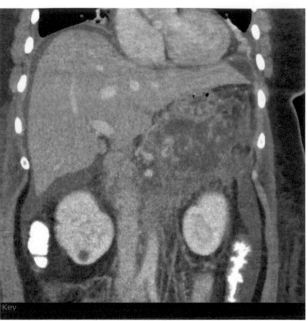

(A) Axial contrast-enhanced computed tomography (CT) shows pancreatic and peripancreatic necrosis with an acute necrotic collection. (B) Coronal contrast-enhanced CT shows pancreatic and peripancreatic necrosis with an acute necrotic collection.

■ **Differential Diagnosis**

- **Acute necrotic collection:** Occurs in the first 4 weeks of acute necrotizing pancreatitis and presents as nonencapsulated peripancreatic or remote fluid.
- *Acute peripancreatic fluid collection:* Occurs in the first 4 weeks of acute interstitial pancreatitis and presents as nonencapsulated peripancreatic fluid.
- *Pseudocyst:* Occurs after the first 4 weeks of acute interstitial pancreatitis and presents as an encapsulated peripancreatic or remote fluid collection with a well-defined wall.
- *Walled-off necrosis:* Occurs after the first 4 weeks of acute necrotizing pancreatitis and presents as encapsulated, nonliquefied tissue with a well-defined wall.

■ **Essential Facts**

- The revised Atlanta Classification for Acute Pancreatitis is based on contrast-enhanced CT findings.
- Necrotizing pancreatitis is categorized based on the tissue undergoing necrosis and is categorized as pancreatic necrosis, peripancreatic necrosis, or pancreatic/peripancreatic necrosis.
- A collection that results from tissue necrosis is termed "acute necrotic collection" in the first 4 weeks. Later in the course when there is encapsulation, the collection is termed "walled-off necrosis."

■ **Other Imaging Findings**

- Magnetic resonance imaging/magnetic resonance cholangiopancreatography is an excellent modality to evaluate pancreatic necrosis. In particular, subtraction of contrast and noncontrast images can accurately detect necrosis.
- Ultrasound can detect peripancreatic fluid collections but may not be able to characterize them.

✓ **Pearls and ✗ Pitfalls**

✓ The onset or duration of pancreatitis is useful in classifying the collections.

✓ Intravenous contrast is essential in determining necrosis.

✓ Gas in the collection without prior intervention is a sign of infection.

✗ Splenic vein and other venous thrombosis may be hard to detect in the presence of the inflammation associated with pancreatitis.

✗ Small pseudoaneurysms may be hard to detect with the inflammation.

Case 33

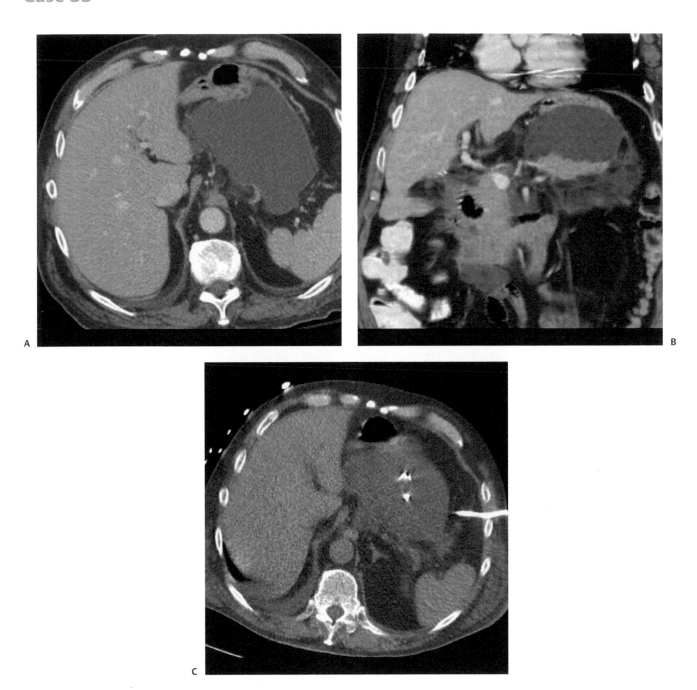

A

B

C

■ **Clinical Presentation**

A 72-year-old-man with resolving pancreatitis (> 4 weeks), now with abdominal fullness.

■ **Imaging Findings**

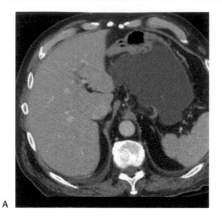 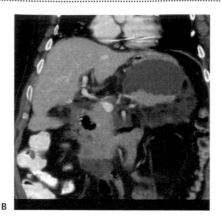 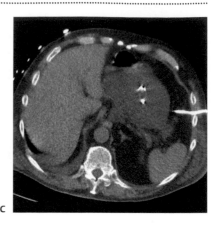

A   B   C

(A) Axial contrast-enhanced computed tomography (CT) shows a well-demarcated fluid collection about the tail of the pancreas. **(B)** Coronal contrast-enhanced CT shows the fluid collection and some residual inflammatory changes around the tail of the pancreas and no pancreatic necrosis. **(C)** Drainage of the fluid collection with placement of a percutaneous drainage catheter.

■ **Differential Diagnosis**

• **Pseudocyst:** Occurs after the first 4 weeks of acute interstitial pancreatitis: encapsulated peripancreatic or remote fluid collections with a well-defined wall.
• *Acute peripancreatic fluid collection:* Occurs in the first 4 weeks of acute interstitial pancreatitis: nonencapsulated peripancreatic fluid collection.
• *Acute necrotic collection:* Occurs in the first 4 weeks of acute necrotizing pancreatitis: nonencapsulated peripancreatic or remote fluid collection.
• *Walled-off necrosis:* Occurs after the first 4 weeks of acute necrotizing pancreatitis: encapsulated, nonliquefied tissue with a well-defined wall.

■ **Essential Facts**

• The revised Atlanta Classification for Acute Pancreatitis is based on contrast-enhanced CT findings.
• A pseudocyst represents evolution of an acute pancreatic fluid collection, occurs 4 weeks after the symptom onset, and is evidenced by the formation of a thickened wall.
• Round or oval homogenous fluid collection surrounded by a well-defined wall with no associated tissue necrosis within the fluid collection.

• Pancreatic necrosis does not evolve into a pseudocyst.
• A total of 50% of pseudocysts will resolve without any intervention, especially if small (< 6 cm) and asymptomatic.
• Pseudocysts can form distant from the pancreas.

■ **Other Imaging Findings**

• At ultrasound, pseudocysts are well-demarcated fluid collections with or without mass effect.
• Magnetic resonance imaging/magnetic resonance cholangiopancreatography is excellent for the evaluation of the pancreas for a pseudocyst. Communication with the pancreatic duct may be demonstrated.

✓ **Pearls and ✗ Pitfalls**

✓ Well-formed pseudocysts can be safely drained.
✓ Gas in a pseudocyst can be a sign of infection.
✗ Pseudocysts can be present in the setting of chronic pancreatitis and should not be mistaken for malignancy.
✗ Injury to the splenic artery and adjacent vessels should be carefully evaluated for pseudoaneurysms.

Case 34

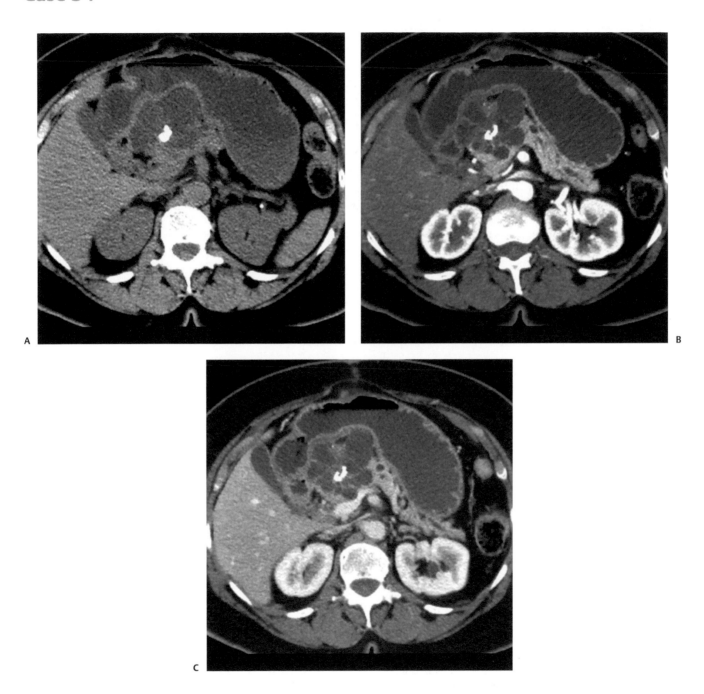

A

B

C

■ Clinical Presentation

A 76-year-old female has a work-up of a pancreatic mass seen on computed tomography (CT).

■ **Imaging Findings**

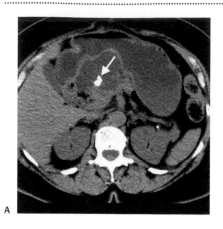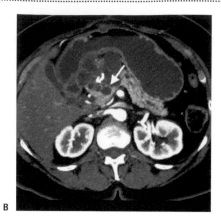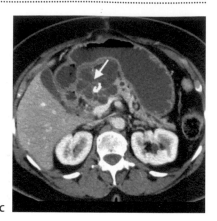

(A) Noncontrast CT shows cystic pancreatic mass with central calcification (*arrow*). **(B)** Arterial phase CT shows some enhancement of the septations of the mass (*arrow*). **(C)** Portal venous phase CT shows enhancement of the septations of the mass (*arrow*).

■ **Differential Diagnosis**

- ***Serous cystadenoma:*** A benign, slow-growing, cystic pancreatic neoplasm that does not communicate with the pancreatic duct.
- *Mucinous cystic neoplasm:* A cystic pancreatic neoplasm that is lined with columnar, mucin-producing epithelium that does not communicate with the pancreatic duct. The malignant potential is variable.
- *Pseudocyst:* Occurs after the first 4 weeks of acute interstitial pancreatitis: encapsulated peripancreatic or remote fluid collection with a well-defined wall.

■ **Essential Facts**

- Serous cystadenoma is a benign lesion that occurs in older women; 80% occur in women over 60 years of age.
- The lesion has a lobular contour made up of multiple small cysts with a thin (< 2 mm) nonenhancing wall.
- Three main types include polycystic (70%), microcystic (20%), and oligocystic (10%).
- Calcifications if present are centrally located.
- Serous cystadenomas can have fibrous radiating septae and localized mass effect.

■ **Other Imaging Findings**

- On magnetic resonance imaging/magnetic resonance cholangiopancreatography, the lesions are T2-hyperintense with T1/T2-hypointense bands and calcification. Communication with the duct cannot be established.

✓ **Pearls and ✗ Pitfalls**

✓ Location in the pancreatic head, a wall thickness of < 2 mm that does not enhance, and a lobular contour are helpful in making the diagnosis.
✓ Central calcification and radiating fibrous bands can be present.
✗ Oligocystic lesions can mimic mucinous tumors.
✗ Lesions can grow and cause ductal obstruction.

Case 35

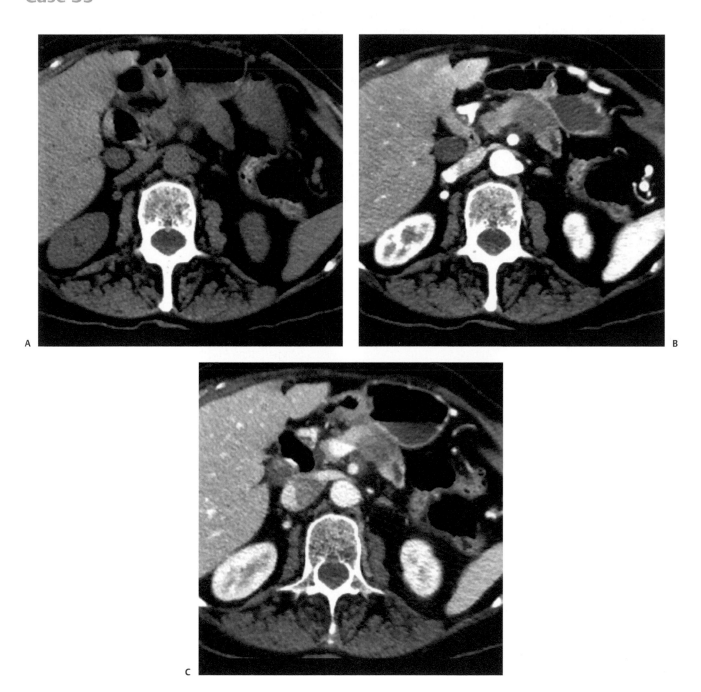

A

B

C

■ Clinical Presentation
....

An 82-year-old female with abdominal pain.

■ **Imaging Findings**

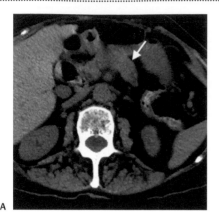 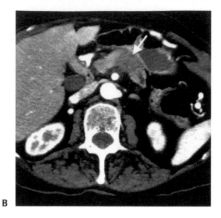 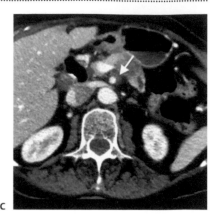

(A) Unenhanced computed tomography (CT) shows an ill-defined mass in the body of the pancreas (*arrow*). (B) Arterial contrast-enhanced CT shows a poorly enhancing mass in the body of the pancreas (*arrow*). (C) Portal venous phase CT shows a poorly enhancing mass in the pancreas with ductal dilation and soft tissue surrounding the proximal branch of the superior mesenteric artery (*arrow*).

■ **Differential Diagnosis**

- **Pancreatic adenocarcinoma:** The most common pancreatic malignancy; derived from adenocarcinoma from pancreatic ductal epithelia.
- *Focal pancreatitis:* Acute pancreatitis that affects a segment of pancreatic parenchyma with surrounding inflammatory changes.

■ **Essential Facts**

- Pancreatic adenocarcinomas can occlude the pancreatic duct when located in the body and can occlude both the pancreatic duct and the common bile duct when in the head, producing the double duct sign.
- The arterial and portal venous phases are used to delineate the mass because normal pancreas enhances vigorously and pancreatic adenocarcinoma is usually comparatively hypoattenuated on contrast-enhanced studies.
- Pancreatic adenocarcinoma is associated with infiltrative growth in the upper abdomen, narrowing or occlusion of vessels, and preferential metastasis to the liver.
- The American Joint Committee on Cancer (AJCC) defines stages I and II as no overt metastatic disease, no overt adenopathy, and, importantly, no evidence of any tumor contact with vasculature. Size-based staging has been used to stratify overall survival.

■ **Other Imaging Findings**

- Magnetic resonance imaging (MRI)/magnetic resonance cholangiopancreatography is useful in diagnosing underlying pancreatic masses. The focal loss of the inherent T1-hyperintensity of the pancreas helps diagnose CT-occult lesions.

✓ **Pearls and ✗ Pitfalls**

- ✓ Evaluation of the upper abdominal vasculature and liver is important in staging.
- ✓ Dilatation of the pancreatic duct or focal pancreatitis should be followed up as this may indicate a small underlying lesion.
- ✗ Approximately 10% of pancreatic adenocarcinomas are isoattenuating to pancreatic parenchyma.
- ✗ Ascites in the upper abdomen can indicate peritoneal involvement.

Case 36

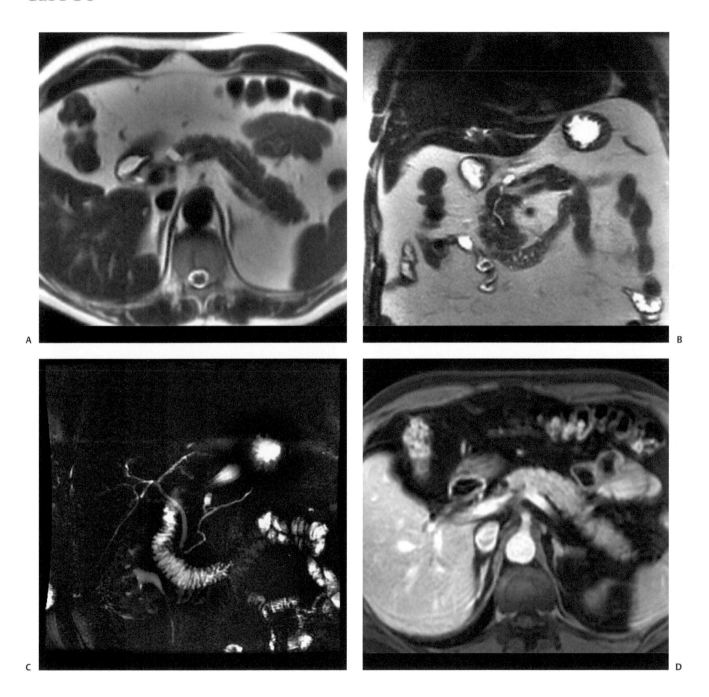

A

B

C

D

■ Clinical Presentation

A 68-year-old female with incidental pancreatic lesion for further evaluation.

■ **Imaging Findings**

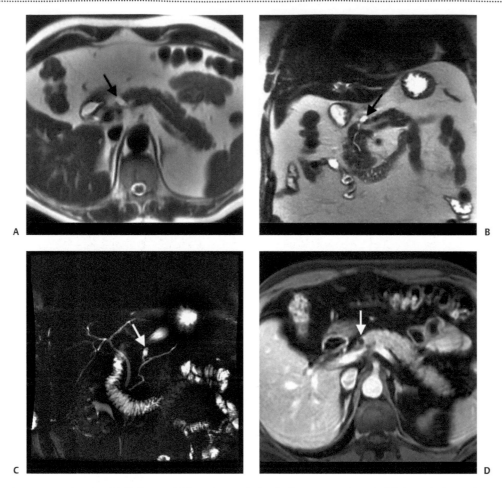

(A) Axial T2 magnetic resonance imaging (MRI) shows a T2-hyperintense lesion in the pancreas (*arrow*). **(B)** Coronal T2 MRI shows a T2-hyperintense lesion in the pancreas (*arrow*). **(C)** Coronal T2 magnetic resonance cholangiopancreatography shows a connection between the lesion and the pancreatic duct (*arrow*). **(D)** Axial postcontrast fast spoiled gradient echo shows no appreciable enhancement in the lesion (*arrow*).

■ **Differential Diagnosis**

- **Side branch intraductal papillary mucinous neoplasm (IPMN) of pancreas:** A cystic, mucin-producing, pancreatic neoplasm that arises in a side branch.
- *Side branch ectasia:* Dilated side branches can be seen in the setting of pancreatitis.
- *Small pseudocyst:* Occurs after the first 4 weeks of acute interstitial pancreatitis: encapsulated peripancreatic or remote fluid collection with a well-defined wall.

■ **Essential Facts**

- IPMNs involve the main pancreatic duct or its major branches and lack associated ovarian-type stroma.
- Rim-like enhancement of the dilated ducts results from compressed or atrophic pancreatic parenchyma replaced by fibrotic tissue.
- Malignancy in a side branch IPMN occurs in 7–34% of cases.

- Nodular enhancement, size > 3 cm, and main duct dilation are predictors of malignancy.
- IPMN occurs in older men; 70% occur in men over 65 years of age.

■ **Other Imaging Findings**

- Computed tomography is useful in staging and can identify IPMNs. Demonstration of connection with the duct may not be feasible.

✓ **Pearls and ✕ Pitfalls**

✓ Demonstration of a connection to the pancreatic duct is important for the diagnosis.
✓ Look for nodular enhancement or wall thickening.
✕ Dilated main branch in the setting of side branch IPMN indicates a combined type and is more likely malignant.
✕ Small cystic lesions such as cystic islet cell tumors may be difficult to distinguish from IPMN.

Case 37

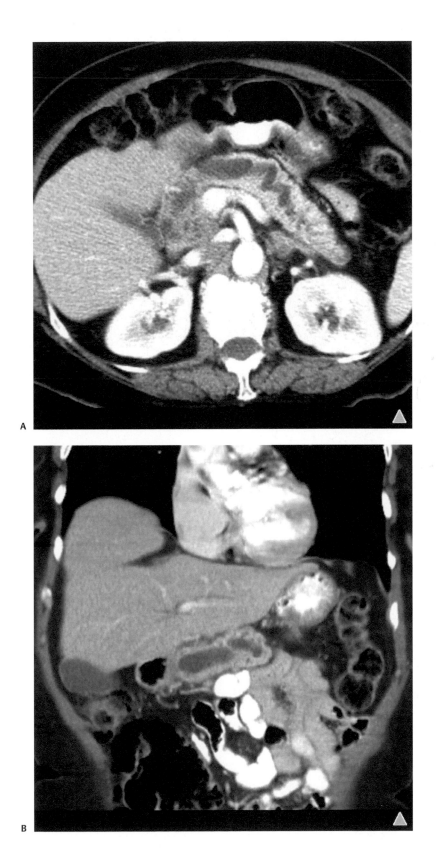

A

B

■ Clinical Presentation

A 78-year-old female with weight loss.

■ **Imaging Findings**

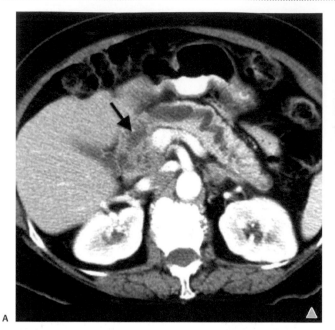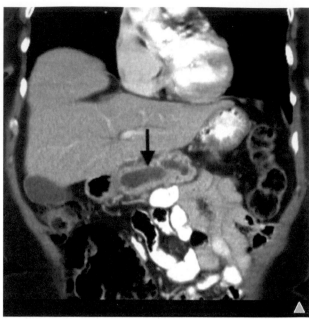

A   B

(A) Axial contrast-enhanced computed tomography (CT) shows a dilated, tortuous main pancreatic duct and a hypoattenuating lesion in the pancreatic head *(arrow)*. **(B)** Coronal contrast-enhanced CT shows the dilated duct and few dilated side branches *(arrow)*.

■ **Differential Diagnosis**

- ***Main branch intraductal papillary mucinous neoplasm (IPMN) of the pancreas:*** Neoplasm originating from mucinous epithelium of the pancreatic duct system and characterized by papillary growth and hyperproduction of mucin, which causes duct dilatation.
- *Pancreatic duct stricture:* Focal or diffuse narrowing of the pancreatic duct caused by either benign or malignant etiologies.

■ **Essential Facts**

- Malignancy can occur as an in situ or invasive cancer in 30–88% of IPMNs with a much higher malignant risk for a main branch compared with a side branch IPMN.
- Mural nodules or main pancreatic duct dilated ≥ 10 mm is highly suggestive of malignancy.
- A dilated duct ≥ 10 mm has a specificity of 92% and sensitivity of 78% for the presence of malignancy.
- Enhancement of the duct wall, dilation of the main duct between 5 and 9 mm, a nonenhancing mural nodule, or focal stenosis and pancreatic atrophy are worrisome features.
- The mucin produced by the lesion causes the major papilla to bulge.

■ **Other Imaging Findings**

- Magnetic resonance imaging/magnetic resonance cholangiopancreatography (MRCP) is the best modality to work up a dilated pancreatic duct. It can demonstrate ductal anatomy, enhancing and nonenhancing nodules, side branch lesions, and ductal wall enhancement.

✓ **Pearls and ✗ Pitfalls**

- ✓ Main pancreatic duct size ≥ 5 mm should be worked up for an underlying lesion using endoscopic ultrasound-guided fine needle aspiration.
- ✓ Focal pancreatic duct stenosis with pancreatic atrophy requires further workup.
- ✗ Benign strictures can cause pancreatic ductal dilation.
- ✗ Focal ductal dilation particularly in the tail can be a sign of a main branch IPMN.

Case 38

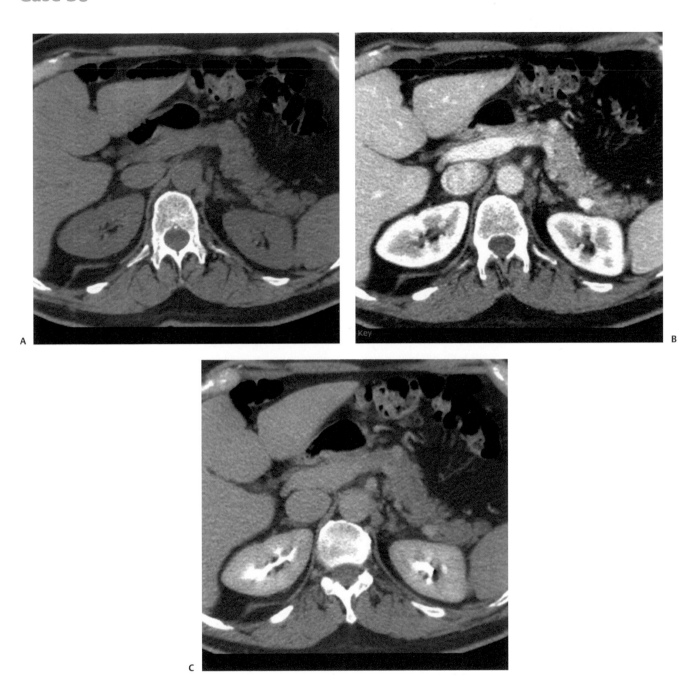

■ **Clinical Presentation**

A 63-year-old male with diarrhea, indigestion, and bloating.

■ Imaging Findings

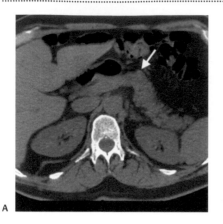 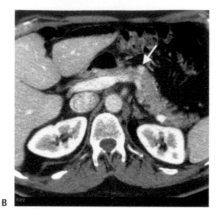 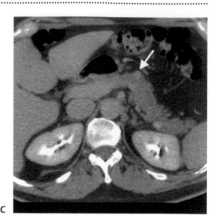

(A) Axial noncontrast computed tomography (CT) of the pancreas shows a focal contour deformity of the pancreatic body (*arrow*). **(B)** Arterial phase CT shows brisk enhancement of the pancreatic body lesion (*arrow*). **(C)** Delayed phase CT shows retention of contrast in the lesion (*arrow*).

■ Differential Diagnosis

- ***Pancreatic neuroendocrine tumor (PNET):*** Arises from the endocrine cells of the pancreas and can be benign or malignant, and hormonally active or nonfunctioning.
- *Metastasis:* Hypervascular metastases to the pancreas commonly include renal cell carcinoma and melanoma.

■ Essential Facts

- PNETs comprise a wide range of endocrine neoplasms that include gastrinoma, insulinoma, glucagonoma, VIPoma, somatostatinoma, and ACTHoma.
- They represent ~8–10% of all pancreatic carcinomas.
- Malignant forms of the lesions can metastasize to the liver, lung, and bones.
- A total of 60% of functioning PNETs are insulinomas. Insulinomas are usually benign whereas other PNETs are often malignant.
- PNETs with a fibrous matrix can produce duct strictures.
- There is an increased incidence of PNETs in syndromes like multiple endocrine neoplasia 1, von Hippel-Lindau, tuberous sclerosis, and neurofibromatosis type 1.

■ Other Imaging Findings

- Magnetic resonance imaging is excellent for evaluating PNETs. They are isointense to muscle on T1-weighted imaging, have moderate to avid enhancement, and are iso- to hyperintense to muscle on T2-weighted imaging. These lesions show restricted diffusion.

✓ Pearls and ✗ Pitfalls

- ✓ Imaging should include an arterial phase as many lesions are hypervascular.
- ✓ Focal ductal narrowing can be caused by a PNET.
- ✗ Some islet cell tumors are cystic and mimic IPMNs but have a hypervascular rim.
- ✗ A total of 50% of functioning islet cell tumors are < 1.3 cm in size.

Case 39

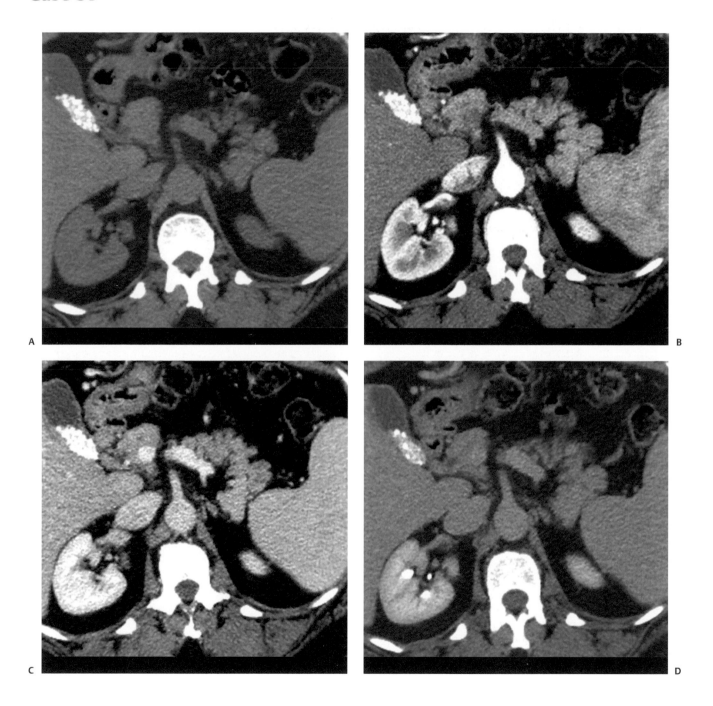

■ **Clinical Presentation**

A 63-year-old male with incidentally detected pancreatic tail mass.

■ Imaging Findings

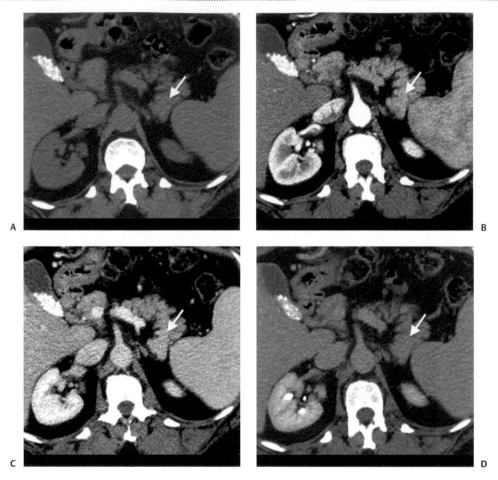

(A) Noncontrast computed tomography (CT) shows subtle enlargement of the pancreatic tail with loss of the parenchymal fat (*arrow*). **(B)** Axial arterial phase CT shows focal enhancement of the pancreatic tail similar to the spleen (*arrow*). **(C)** Axial portal venous phase CT shows focal enhancement of the pancreatic tail similar to the spleen (*arrow*). **(D)** Delayed phase CT shows the pancreatic tail with similar enhancement as the spleen (*arrow*).

■ Differential Diagnosis

- ***Intrapancreatic accessory spleen (IPAS):*** Accessory spleen is a congenital abnormality consisting of normal splenic tissue in ectopic sites.
- *Pancreatic neuroendocrine neoplasm:* Arises from the endocrine cells of the pancreas and can be benign or malignant, or hormonally active or nonfunctioning.

■ Essential Facts

- Accessory spleen forms from congenital splenic tissue outside the spleen and results from failure of fusion of some of the multiple buds of splenic tissue in the dorsal mesogastrium during embryologic life.
- The second most common site is the tail of the pancreas after the inferior portion of the splenic hilum.
- Accessory spleen is almost never present lateral or superior to the spleen.
- The tissue should appear identical to the spleen in all sequences and phases of contrast administration.

■ Other Imaging Findings

- Technetium-99m–labeled heat-damaged red blood cell scintigraphy with single-photon emission CT imaging can be used to confirm splenic tissue.

✓ Pearls and ✗ Pitfalls

- ✓ Pathology that involves the spleen also tends to involve the accessory spleen.
- ✓ A draining vein can sometimes be identified that drains into the splenic vein.
- ✗ IPAS can mimic a neuroendocrine neoplasm.
- ✗ A single-phase CT may not be able to adequately characterize the lesion.

Case 40

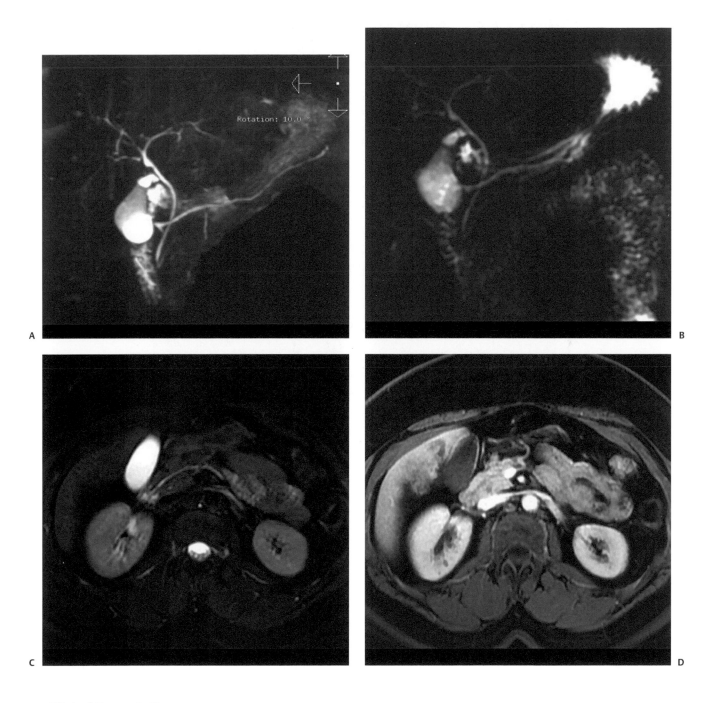

A

B

C

D

■ Clinical Presentation

A 54-year-old female with chronic abdominal pain.

■ **Imaging Findings**

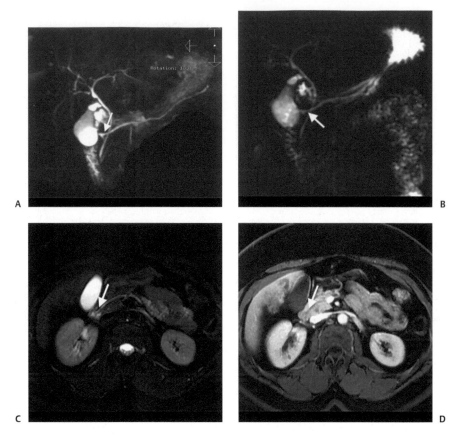

(A) Coronal maximum intensity projection magnetic resonance cholangiopancreatography (MRCP) shows the main pancreatic duct (MPD) draining into the duodenum via the minor papilla (Santorini) (*arrow*). **(B)** Coronal T2 MRCP shows the MPD crossing anterior to the common bile duct (CBD) (*arrow*). **(C)** Axial T2 shows the MPD crossing the CBD to drain via the minor papilla (*arrow*). **(D)** Postcontrast T1-spoiled gradient imaging shows the MPD crossing over the CBD (*arrow*).

■ **Differential Diagnosis**

- ***Pancreas divisum:*** A pancreatic ductal abnormality where a small ventral duct drains through the larger major papilla and the larger dorsal duct drains through the smaller minor papilla.
- *Incomplete pancreas divisum:* A bifid duct where the larger dorsal duct drains through the smaller minor papilla but has a connection to the smaller ventral duct that drains through the larger major papilla.

■ **Essential Facts**

- Pancreas divisum is a congenital abnormality formed from the failure of fusion of the ventral and dorsal pancreatic buds.
- The main pancreatic duct drains via the minor papilla into the duodenum.
- It occurs in ~14% of individuals.
- It may cause pain and acute pancreatitis.

■ **Other Imaging Findings**

- On computed tomography (CT), the diagnosis of divisum may be established if the ducts are dilated.
- Endoscopic retrograde cholangiopancreatography (ERCP) is an invasive alternative to MRCP to evaluate pancreatic ductal anatomy.

✓ **Pearls and** ✗ **Pitfalls**

- ✓ MRCP is modality of choice to noninvasively evaluate the ductal anatomy.
- ✓ Secretin administration helps distend the duct for better visualization.
- ✗ The presence of acute inflammation can obscure the pancreatic ductal anatomy.
- ✗ Ducts that are tortuous can be difficult to evaluate.

Case 41

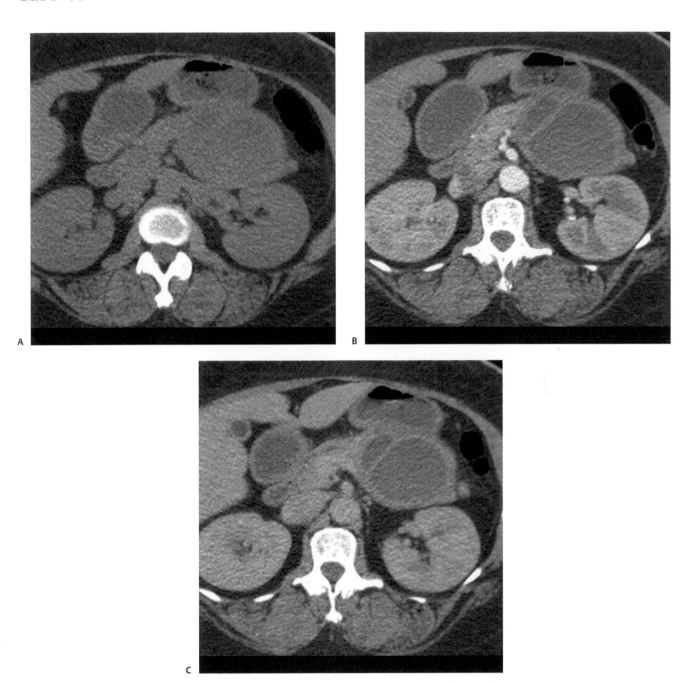

A

B

C

■ Clinical Presentation

A 56-year-old female with a pancreatic mass for work-up.

■ **Imaging Findings**

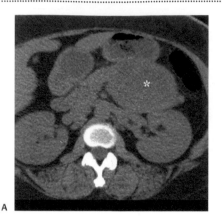 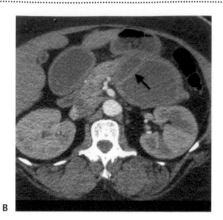 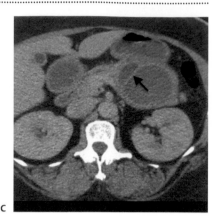

A   B   C

(A) Noncontrast computed tomography (CT) shows a pancreatic tail mass (*asterisk*). **(B)** Contrast-enhanced portal venous CT shows a cystic mass in the pancreatic tail with a thick septation and wall enhancement (*arrow*). **(C)** Delayed phase CT shows the cystic mass without enhancement of the cystic portion (*arrow*).

■ **Differential Diagnosis**

• ***Mucinous cystadenoma:*** A mucinous cystic epithelial neoplasm considered benign but sometimes indistinguishable by imaging from a malignant lesion.
• *Pseudocyst:* Occurs after the first 4 weeks of acute interstitial pancreatitis: encapsulated peripancreatic or remote fluid collection with a well-defined wall.

■ **Essential Facts**

• Mucinous cystic neoplasm can be one of the following: benign mucinous cystadenoma (72%), borderline mucinous cystic tumor (10.5%), mucinous cystic tumor with carcinoma in situ (5.5%), and, the most aggressive form, mucinous cystadenocarcinoma (12%).
• The majority occur in women (99.7%), most commonly of middle age.
• The lesions most commonly occur in the tail of the pancreas.
• They are round or oval in shape and contain ovarian stroma, histologically.

• They typically do not communicate with the duct.
• The presence of septations, calcifications, and a thick enhancing wall are findings of malignancy.

■ **Other Imaging Findings**

• Magnetic resonance imaging (MRI) shows the lesion as a unilocular or mildly septated cystic lesion.
• MRI may be more sensitive to detect internal enhancing components.

✓ **Pearls and** ✗ **Pitfalls**

✓ Mucinous lesions can be large (> 10 cm) before being detected.
✓ All lesions are considered surgical.
✗ Mucinous tumors can mimic well-formed pseudocysts.
✗ Different portions of the lesion wall may have different degrees of malignant change.

Case 42

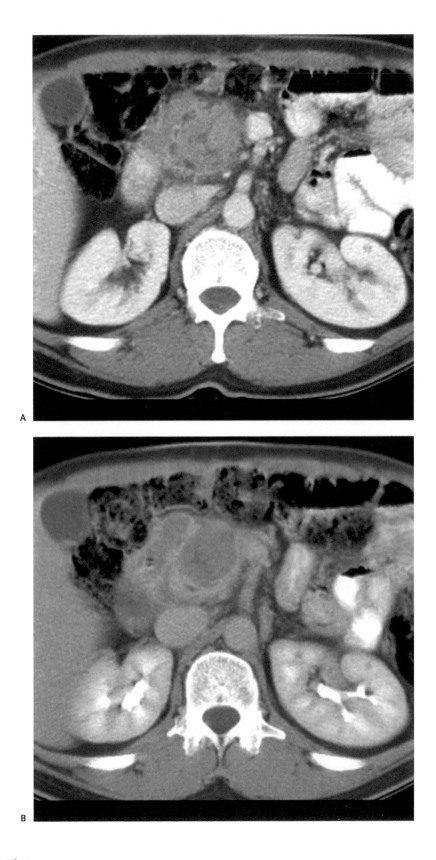

A

B

■ Clinical Presentation

A 55-year-old male with a pancreatic head mass.

■ **Imaging Findings**

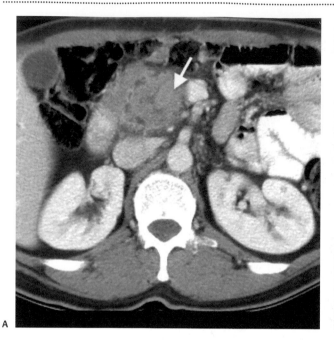 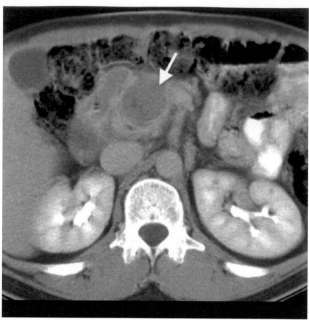

(A) Portal venous phase computed tomography (CT) shows a large solid exophytic mass in the pancreatic head (*arrow*). **(B)** Delayed phase CT shows washout and some capsular enhancement (*arrow*).

■ **Differential Diagnosis**

- *Acinar cell carcinoma:* A rare pancreatic neoplasm that arises from the pancreatic acinar cells.
- *Pancreatic neuroendocrine neoplasm:* Arises from the endocrine cells of the pancreas and can be benign or malignant, and hormonally active or nonfunctioning.

■ **Essential Facts**

- It is a rare tumor of the pancreas arising from acinar cells and comprising 1% of pancreatic neoplasms.
- It is more common in men over the age of 50 years.
- It is commonly exophytic, which is distinctive to the lesion.
- It can be cystic/necrotic or solid.
- Reported cases do not have calcifications.
- Enhancing capsule is common.

■ **Other Imaging Findings**

- On magnetic resonance imaging, the solid lesion can be mildly T2-hyperintense and can mildly enhance.

✓ **Pearls and ✗ Pitfalls**

- ✓ Rare tumor may require biopsy for diagnosis.
- ✓ It can be present in the pancreatic head/uncinate, body, or tail.
- ✗ Some have infiltrative features and can be mistaken for adenocarcinoma.
- ✗ Necrotic lesions may be mistaken for a mucinous neoplasm.

Case 43

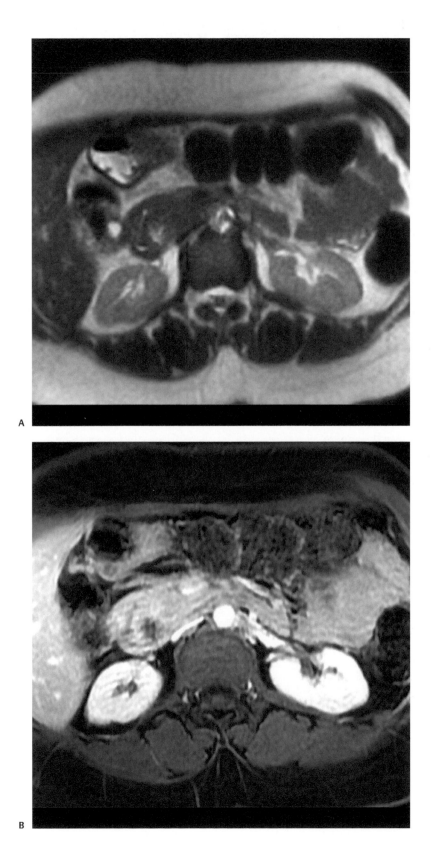

A

B

■ Clinical Presentation

A 47-year-old female with nausea and early satiety.

■ Imaging Findings

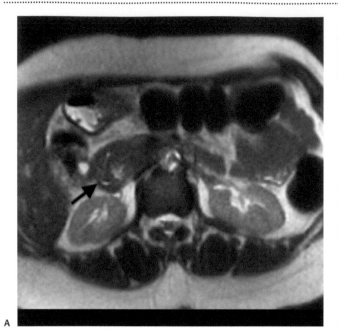 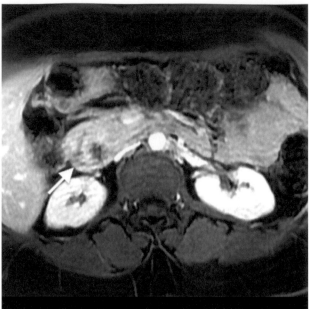

A   B

(A) Axial T2 shows an enlarged pancreatic head with a duct that encircles the duodenum (*arrow*). **(B)** Postcontrast T1-fast spoiled gradient echo shows normal pancreas parenchyma encircling the duodenum (*arrow*).

■ Differential Diagnosis

• ***Annular pancreas:*** Congenital anomaly with pancreatic tissue encircling the duodenum.

■ Essential Facts

• Annular pancreas is a rare congenital anomaly caused by incomplete rotation of the ventral anlage with the duodenum.
• It can be complete or partial, but always demonstrates continuity with the pancreatic head.
• Annular pancreatic duct usually communicates with the main pancreatic duct (MPD) (extramural type) the duct of Wirsung, or the duct of Santorini.
• The second portion of the duodenum is circumferentially narrowed.
• About 50% of patients are asymptomatic.

■ Other Imaging Findings

• Annular pancreas can be detected on computed tomography as circumferential pancreatic tissue around the duodenum.
• Narrowing of the second portion of the duodenum on an upper gastrointestinal barium study should prompt further work-up for annular pancreas or a mass.

✓ Pearls and ✗ Pitfalls

✓ The use of secretin can facilitate better visualization of the pancreatic duct on imaging studies.
✓ Annular pancreas can cause symptomatic duodenal narrowing.
✗ Duodenal narrowing produced by an annular pancreas must not be mistaken for a malignancy.
✗ The pancreatic duct may not drain into the MPD in the intramural type; instead, small ducts directly penetrate the duodenum.

Case 44

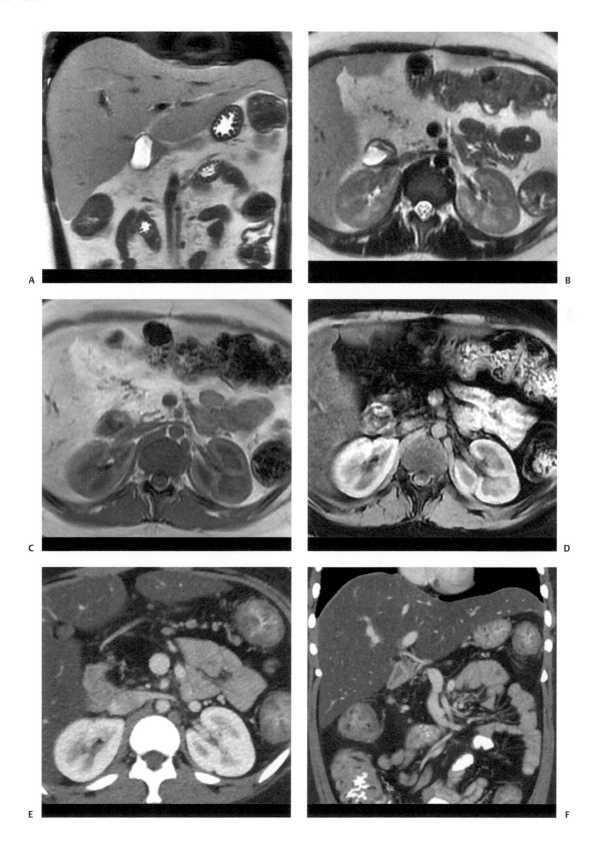

A 20-year-old female with pancreatic insufficiency and elevated liver enzymes.

■ **Imaging Findings**

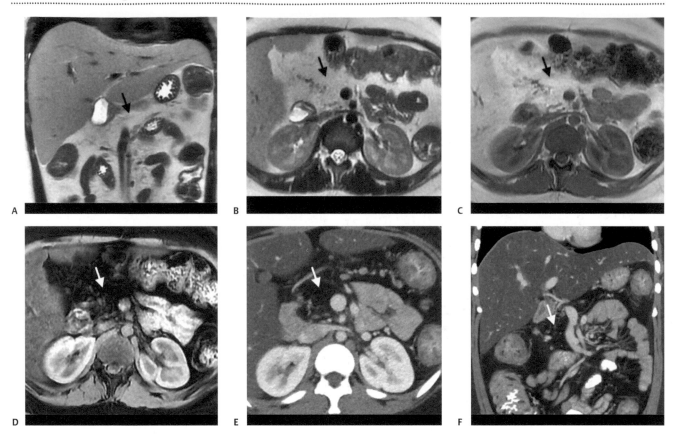

(A) Coronal T2 shows fatty changes in the pancreas (*arrow*). **(B)** Axial T2 shows fatty changes in the pancreas (*arrow*). **(C)** Axial T1 shows complete fatty replacement of the pancreas (*arrow*). **(D)** Axial T1 fat-saturated imaging shows complete fatty replacement of the pancreas with fat suppression of the fatty tissue (*arrow*). **(E)** Axial computed tomography (CT) shows complete fatty replacement of the pancreas (*arrow*). **(F)** Coronal CT shows complete fatty replacement of the pancreas (*arrow*).

■ **Differential Diagnosis**

• ***Pancreatic lipomatosis:*** Fatty infiltration or replacement of the pancreas.
• *Pancreatic atrophy:* Atrophy of the pancreatic parenchyma.
• *Agenesis of the pancreas:* Agenesis of the pancreas is a lethal condition.

■ **Essential Facts**

• Pancreatic lipomatosis is replacement of the pancreatic parenchyma by fat, which occurs in patients with diabetes, cystic fibrosis, Shwachman-Diamond syndrome, Johanson-Blizzard syndrome, and obesity.
• There are four types of distribution of pancreatic lipomatosis: type 1a (35%) is fatty replacement of the head with sparing of the uncinate process and peribiliary region; type 1b (36%) is fatty replacement of the head, neck, and body with sparing of the uncinate process and peribiliary region; type 2a (12%) is fatty replacement of the head, including the uncinate process, and sparing

of the peribiliary region; and type 2b (18%) is fatty total replacement of the pancreas with sparing of the peribiliary region.
• Pancreatic lipomatosis can result in pancreatic insufficiency.

■ **Other Imaging Findings**

• Fatty pancreas on ultrasound shows increased echogenicity.

✓ **Pearls and ✗ Pitfalls**

✓ Fatty replacement of the pancreas can be focal or diffuse.
✓ Fatty replacement of the pancreas can be associated with pancreatic insufficiency.
✗ In cases of pancreatic atrophy, the parenchyma should be evaluated for a mass.
✗ Focal pancreatic fatty infiltration may mimic a mass.

Case 45

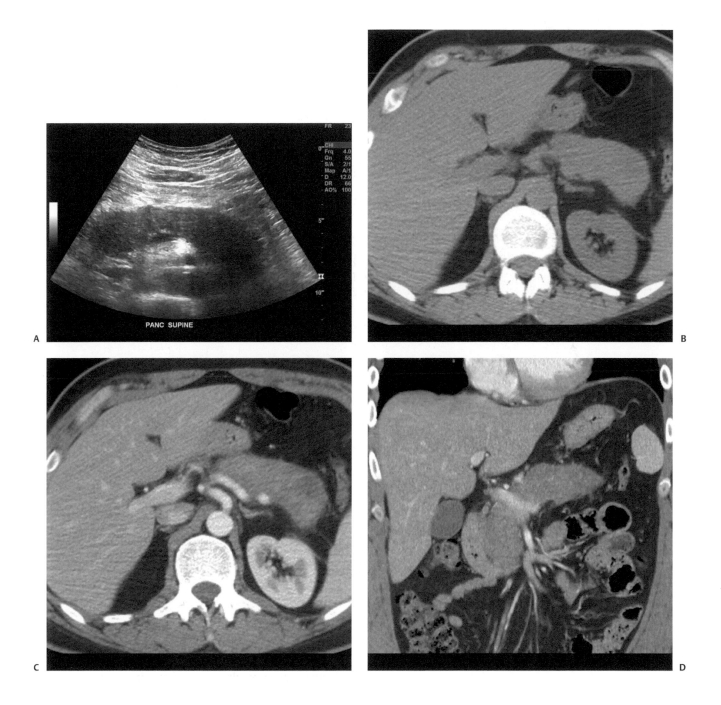

■ Clinical Presentation

A 40-year-old male with chronic abdominal pain and weight loss.

■ **Imaging Findings**

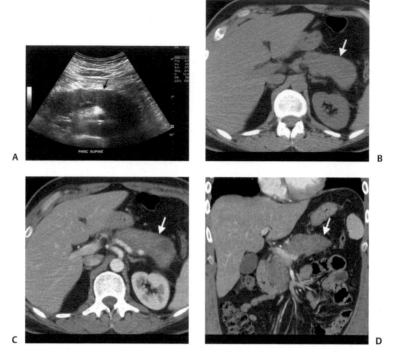

(A) Transabdominal ultrasound of the pancreas shows a hypoechoic, enlarged pancreas without much peripancreatic fluid (*arrow*). **(B)** Axial noncontrast computed tomography (CT) shows an enlarged pancreas, but the peripancreatic fat planes are normal (*arrow*). **(C)** Axial contrast-enhanced CT shows an enlarged pancreas with some inflammation but no surrounding fluid (*arrow*). Subtle hypodensity is present in the tail of the pancreas. **(D)** Coronal contrast-enhanced CT shows an enlarged pancreas with no significant peripancreatic fluid (*arrow*).

■ **Differential Diagnosis**

• **Autoimmune pancreatitis (AIP):** Rare form of chronic pancreatitis secondary to an immune-mediated, fibroinflammatory process associated with elevated serum immunoglobulin 4 (IgG4).
• *Acute interstitial pancreatitis:* Acute inflammation of the pancreas resulting in edema and inflammation of the pancreas.

■ **Essential Facts**

• AIP is a part of a spectrum of IgG4-related diseases of which there are two subtypes:
  ○ AIP type 1: Manifestation of a systemic IgG4-related disease with involvement of other organs such as the salivary glands, bile ducts, and kidneys. Affects older (sixth decade) males and can have elevated serum IgG4. Histology shows IgG4-rich periductal lymphoplasmacytic infiltrates in the pancreas.
  ○ AIP type 2: Is not associated with IgG4 disease. Affects younger patients, both male and female (fourth decade). Histology shows granulocyte epithelial lesions in the pancreas. AIP-2 has an association with chronic inflammatory bowel disease.
• CT shows an enlarged pancreas sometimes with a hypodense halo and no surrounding fat infiltration.

• The pancreas shows delayed enhancement, and the pancreatic duct may enhance.
• It may present with biliary obstruction and lesions in the kidneys.

■ **Other Imaging Findings**

• On magnetic resonance imaging (MRI), the pancreatic parenchyma is T1-hypointense and T2-hyperintense in signal.
• The peripancreatic capsule is hypointense on both T1- and T2-weighted imaging and can have delayed enhancement after contrast administration.
• Magnetic resonance cholangiopancreatography (MRCP) may show ductal dilation in the pancreas and obstruction or narrowing of the biliary ducts.

✓ **Pearls and** ✗ **Pitfalls**

✓ AIP should be suspected in patients with an enlarged pancreas and no surrounding inflammation.
✓ Response to corticosteroids can help establish the diagnosis.
✗ AIP can mimic a pancreatic adenocarcinoma, especially in cases of ductal obstruction.
✗ Diagnosis may be inconclusive on biopsy.

Case 46

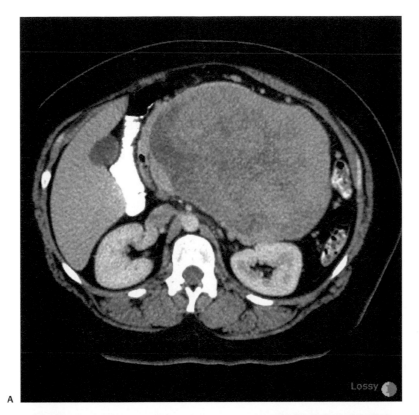

A

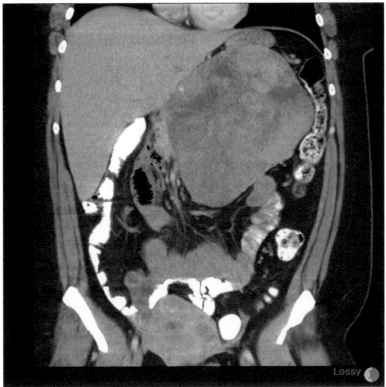

B

■ Clinical Presentation

A 43-year-old female with pancreatic tail mass.

■ **Imaging Findings**

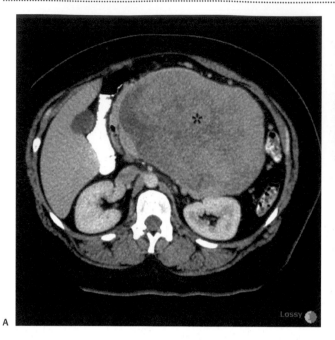
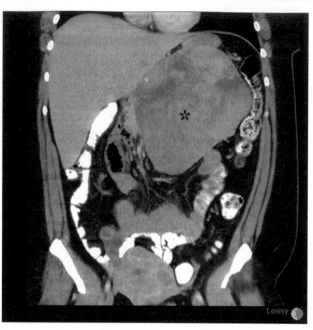

Axial **(A)** and coronal **(B)** contrast-enhanced computed tomography of the abdomen shows a large, solid mass in the tail of the pancreas without any infiltrative features (*asterisks*). Low attenuation areas in the mass are suggestive of necrosis.

■ **Differential Diagnosis**

- ***Solid and papillary epithelial neoplasm (SPEN) of the pancreas:*** Rare pancreatic tumor with low malignant potential that typically occurs in young females.
- *Pancreatic neuroendocrine tumor:* Arises from the endocrine cells of the pancreas and can be benign and malignant, or hormonally active or nonfunctioning.

■ **Essential Facts**

- SPENs typically occur in young women in the second or third decade of life.
- They can be large at presentation.
- They are well-encapsulated with both solid and cystic areas and hemorrhage. The presence of a fibrous capsule can suggest the diagnosis.
- Lesions can have peripheral calcification.
- Histology of the lesion shows solid, pseudopapillary, and cystic changes merging with one another.

■ **Other Imaging Findings**

- On magnetic resonance imaging, the mass is heterogeneous, T1-hypointense, and T2-hyperintense, and can have areas of hemorrhage, necrosis, and cystic change.

✓ **Pearls and** ✗ **Pitfalls**

- ✓ SPENs may metastasize to the liver.
- ✓ Lesions that have delayed enhancement are considered more aggressive.
- ✗ Large lesions may undergo extensive hemorrhage mimicking a cystic pancreatic mass.
- ✗ The presence of calcification is not specific to the entity and can be seen in many other pancreatic neoplasms.

Case 47

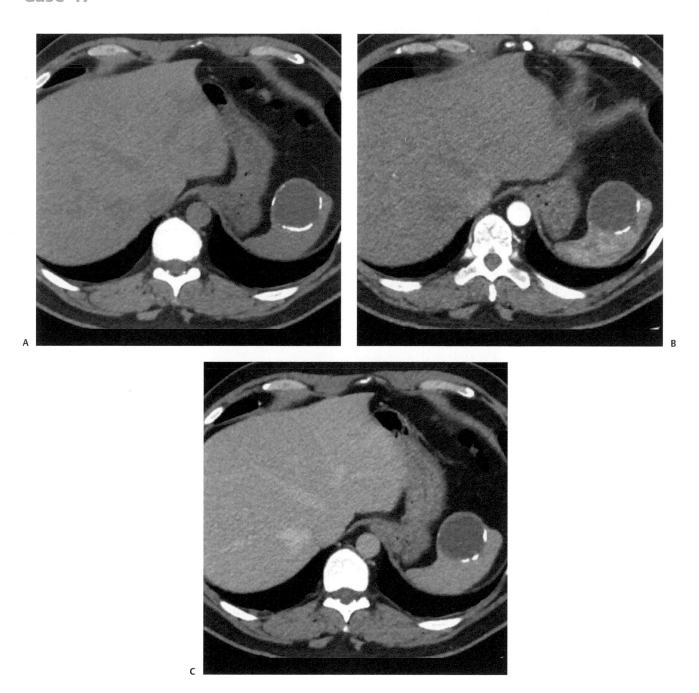

A

B

C

■ Clinical Presentation

A 43-year-old male with a splenic mass.

■ Imaging Findings

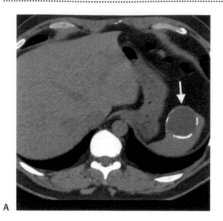 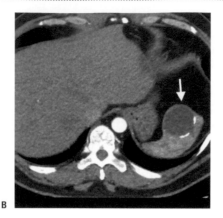 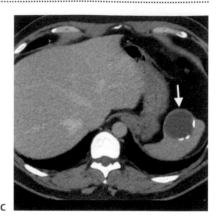

(A) Axial unenhanced computed tomography (CT) shows a peripherally calcified mass in the spleen (*arrow*). **(B)** Axial arterial phase CT shows no arterial enhancement (*arrow*). **(C)** Axial portal venous phase CT shows midlevel enhancement of the fibrous portions of the cyst (*arrow*).

■ Differential Diagnosis

- ***Calcified splenic pseudocyst (secondary):*** Develops after splenic trauma or infection and lacks an epithelial lining.
- *Echinococcal disease (primary): Echinococcus granulosus* causes peripherally calcified splenic and abdominal cystic lesions.
- *Congenital splenic cyst (primary):* A true cyst (epithelial, transitional, or mesothelial); the majority are epidermoid in origin.

■ Essential Facts

- Calcified splenic cysts are secondary and are lined by a fibrous capsule with wall calcifications.
- On CT, they are sharply demarcated, unilocular, low-density lesions without any enhancement.
- They are thought to be the final stage in evolution of a splenic hematoma.
- They can be variable in size.
- They may cause mass effect or hemorrhage which are indications for surgery.

■ Other Imaging Findings

- Magnetic resonance imaging shows the calcified wall as T1- and T2-hypointense. The content of the cyst affects the T1 and T2 signal of the fluid. Cysts lack septations or trabeculae.

✓ Pearls and ✗ Pitfalls

- ✓ Contrast-enhanced study can show that there are no enhancing parts of the lesion.
- ✓ Calcified cysts in other parts of the abdomen may indicate Echinococcal disease.
- ✗ Large intrasplenic aneurysms can mimic secondary cysts.
- ✗ Biopsy is not recommended as this may cause bleeding.

Case 48

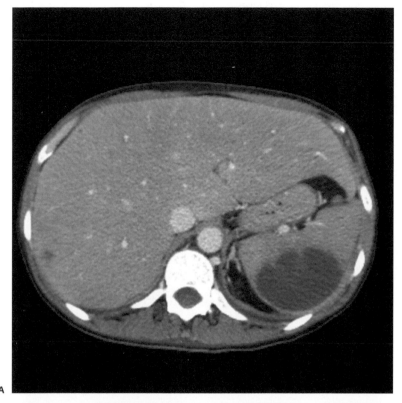

A

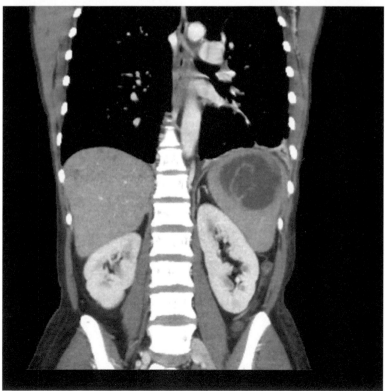

B

■ Clinical Presentation

A 50-year-old immunosuppressed female with fever and pain.

■ **Imaging Findings**

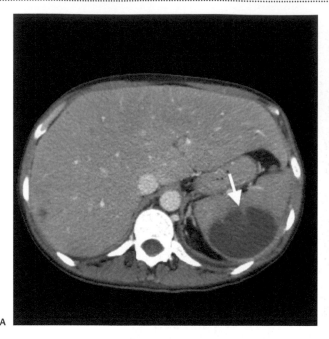 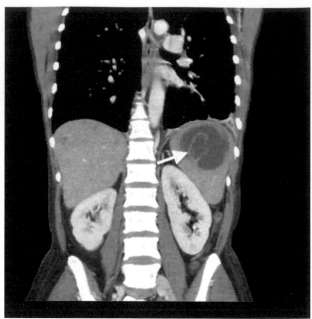

(A) Axial contrast-enhanced computed tomography (CT) shows a splenic cystic lesion with a subtle wall and some surrounding perfusion changes (*arrow*).
(B) Coronal contrast-enhanced CT shows the splenic lesion with thick internal septae and no calcifications (*arrow*).

■ **Differential Diagnosis**

- **Splenic abscess:** Infected collection in the spleen that can be cystic or solid, and solitary or multiple.
- *Calcified splenic pseudocyst (secondary):* Develops after splenic trauma or infection and lacks an epithelial lining.
- *Congenital cyst (primary):* A true cyst that can be epithelial, transitional, or mesothelial.
- *Cystic metastasis:* Treated or necrotic metastasis to the spleen that can be cystic.

■ **Essential Facts**

- Splenic abscess has a high mortality rate of 20–60%.
- Bacterial splenic abscesses can be solitary, multiple, or multiloculated.
- Bacterial abscess is centrally necrotic with an enhancing wall and septae varying in thickness from 1 to 10 mm.
- The presence of gas is diagnostic but is rarely present.
- The combination of immunocompromise and multiple splenic lesions is most suggestive of fungal abscess.

■ **Other Imaging Findings**

- On magnetic resonance imaging, bacterial abscesses are T2-hyperintense, T1-hypointense, can have internal debris, and demonstrate minimal peripheral enhancement when they develop a wall. They tend to restrict diffusion and are hyperintense on diffusion and hypointense on apparent diffusion coefficient maps.

✓ **Pearls and ✗ Pitfalls**

✓ The abscess can be wedge-shaped in patients with bacterial endocarditis and septic emboli.
✓ Contrast-enhanced CT is preferred to make the diagnosis.
✗ Metastatic disease from sources such as lymphoma and melanoma can mimic fungal abscess.
✗ Sarcoid, which is neither malignant nor infectious, can mimic splenic infection.

Case 49

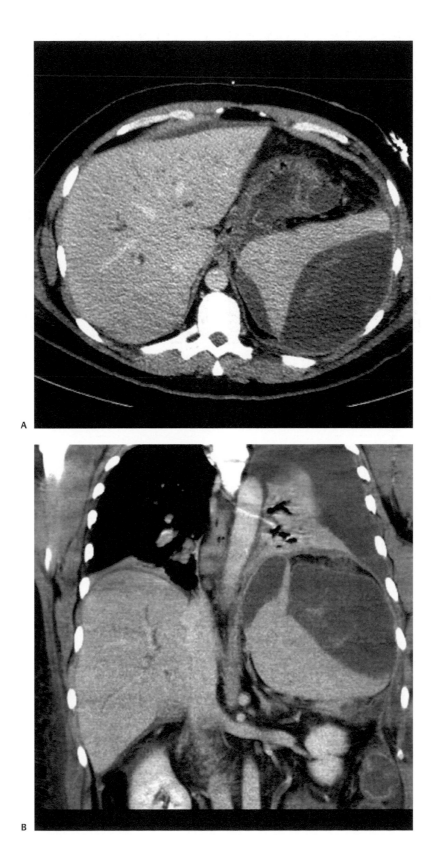

A

B

■ Clinical Presentation

A 56-year-old with left upper quadrant pain.

■ **Imaging Findings**

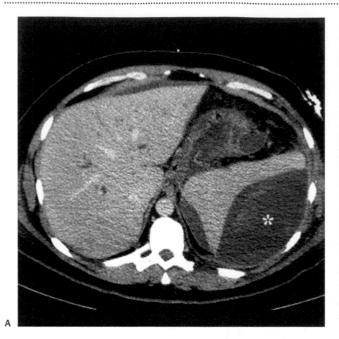
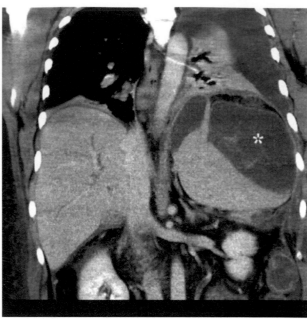

A   B

(A) Axial contrast-enhanced computed tomography (CT) shows a hypodense collection in the subcapsular region with internal heterogeneity from evolving subacute to chronic hematoma (*asterisk*). **(B)** Coronal contrast-enhanced CT shows internal hyperdensity and some septations (*asterisk*).

■ **Differential Diagnosis**

- ***Subcapsular hematoma:*** An intrasplenic hematoma that is contained or partially contained by the capsule.
- *Splenic abscess:* Infected collection in the spleen that can be cystic or solid, and solitary or multiple.
- *Calcified splenic pseudocyst (secondary):* Develops after splenic trauma or infection and lacks an epithelial lining.
- *Congenital cyst (primary):* A true cyst that can be epithelial, transitional, or mesothelial.

■ **Essential Facts**

- Splenic hematomas can result from trauma, iatrogenic injury, and pancreatitis.
- Spontaneous hematoma of the spleen has been reported in drug use.
- Splenic hematomas can rupture and cause left upper quadrant pain (radiates to left shoulder), abdominal hemorrhage, and even death.

■ **Other Imaging Findings**

- On magnetic resonance imaging, splenic hematomas are variable intensity on T1- and T2-weighted imaging with hemorrhage appearing T1-hyperintense.

✓ **Pearls and ✗ Pitfalls**

✓ Subcapsular hematomas should be evaluated for an underlying cause and ongoing hemorrhage/ hemoperitoneum.
✓ Hematomas may require splenic artery embolization.
✗ Subcapsular hematomas can become infected.
✗ Biopsy of the hematoma can cause hemorrhage.

Case 50

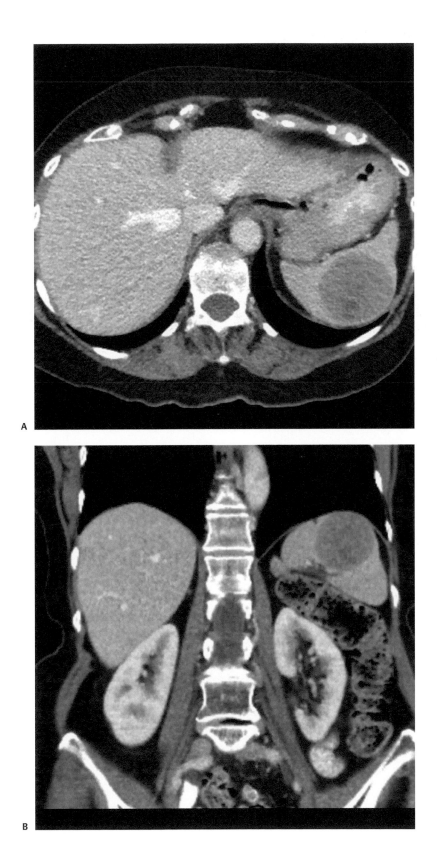

A

B

■ Clinical Presentation

A 70-year-old female with screening computed tomography (CT).

■ **Imaging Findings**

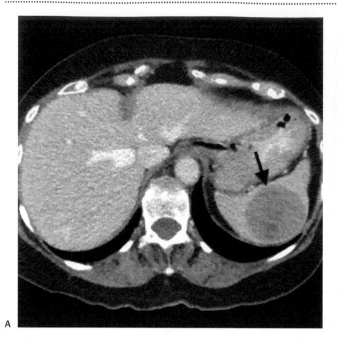 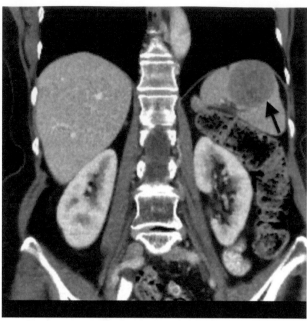

A   B

Axial **(A)** and coronal **(B)** contrast-enhanced CT shows a solid mass in the spleen that is hypoenhancing relative to background spleen (*arrows*).

■ **Differential Diagnosis**

- ***Splenic metastasis:*** Splenic metastasis is rare; however, certain malignancies have an increased risk of splenic involvement.
- *Primary splenic lesions:* Benign hamartomas, intermediate lesions, hemangioendotheliomas, hemangiopericytomas, littoral cell angiomas, and malignant hemangiosarcomas.

■ **Essential Facts**

- Splenic metastasis is rare, seen in 2–9% of untreated cancer patients.
- Breast, lung, colon, ovary, stomach, melanoma, pancreas, cervix, liver, and lymphoma most commonly metastasize to the spleen.
- Isolated splenic metastasis can be seen in up to 5% of patients with a malignancy.

■ **Other Imaging Findings**

- On magnetic resonance imaging, the lesions are intermediate on T2 and show enhancement. They can restrict diffusion.

✓ **Pearls and ✗ Pitfalls**

- ✓ Lesions that are new in the setting or a malignancy are suspicious for metastasis.
- ✓ Lesions that enhance less than splenic parenchyma are considered solid splenic lesions.
- ✗ Splenic involvement may be the only site of metastasis.
- ✗ Splenic lesions can be hard to detect on earlier phases of imaging.

Case 51

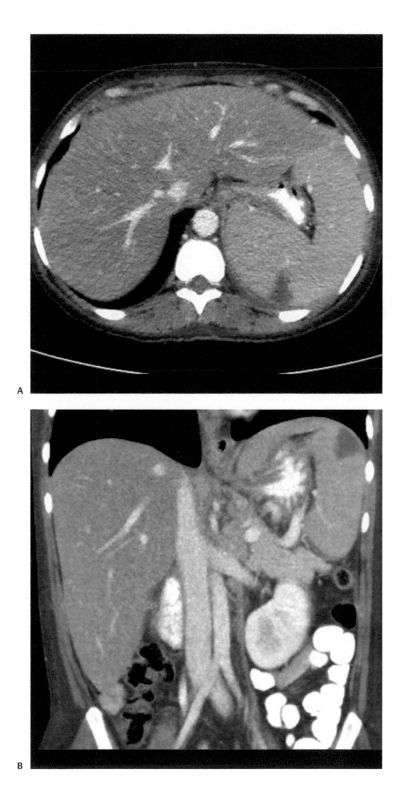

A

B

■ Clinical Presentation

A 44-year-old with elevated lactate and persistent tachycardia.

■ **Imaging Findings**

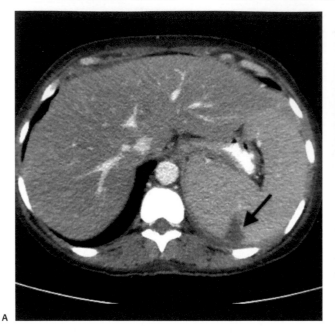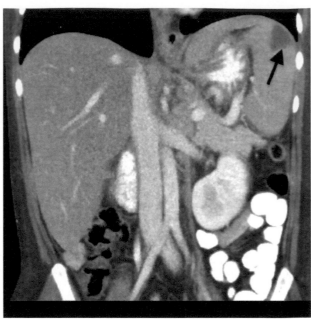

A   B

(A) Axial contrast-enhanced computed tomography (CT) shows a peripheral, wedge-shaped area of hypoperfusion in an enlarged spleen (*arrow*). **(B)** Coronal contrast-enhanced CT shows the wedge-shaped area extending to the capsule (*arrow*). Note there is no surrounding hematoma.

■ **Differential Diagnosis**

- **Splenic infarction:** Result of splenic ischemia causing areas of decreased perfusion.
- **Splenic laceration:** Traumatic injury to the spleen resulting in a parenchymal defect.

■ **Essential Facts**

- Causes of splenic infarction include thromboembolic disease, infiltrative hematologic diseases, hypercoagulable states, pancreatitis, and trauma.
- Splenic infarctions can cause left upper quadrant abdominal pain.
- Chronically, they appear as areas of scarring.
- Treatment is focused on treating the underlying cause.

■ **Other Imaging Findings**

- On ultrasound, splenic infarctions are hypoechoic, peripherally located, and can be wedge-shaped or rounded.

✓ **Pearls and** ✗ **Pitfalls**

- ✓ The infarcted segment can be wedge-shaped, round, or irregular.
- ✓ Splenic infarctions are best evaluated in the portal venous phase when the splenic parenchyma has uniform enhancement.
- ✗ Peripheral splenic lacerations can have a linear appearance that may mimic an infarction.
- ✗ Thromboembolic disease most commonly results from cardiac disease and can cause other organ infarctions in addition to splenic infarction.

Case 52

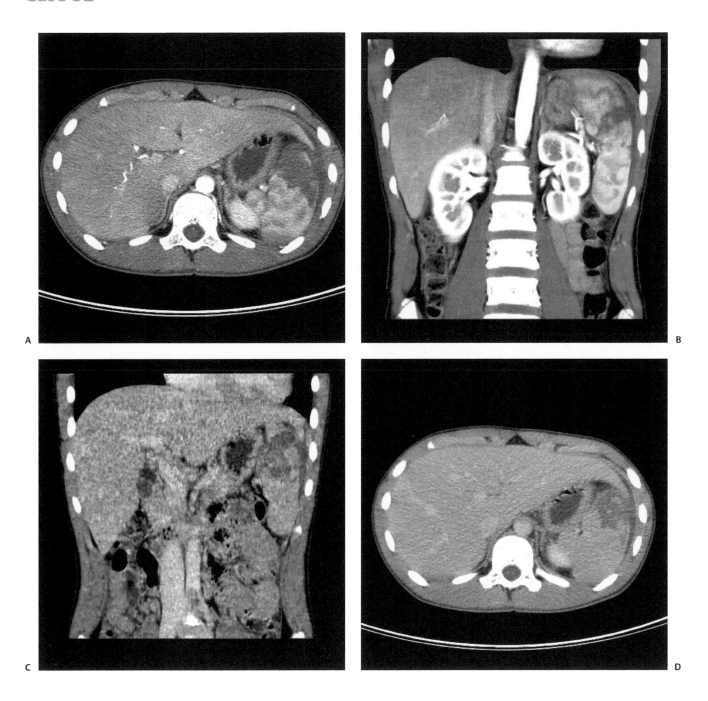

A

B

C

D

■ Clinical Presentation

A 24-year-old male with abdominal pain after trauma and + focused assessment with sonography for trauma scan.

■ Imaging Findings

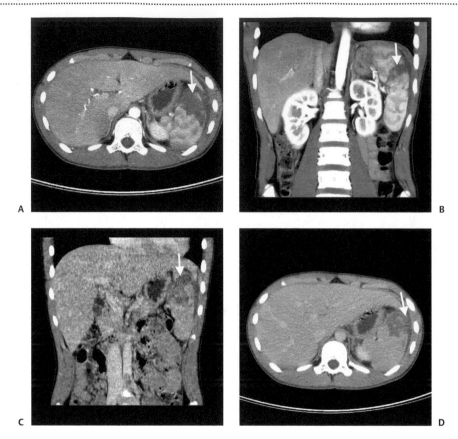

(A) Axial, arterial phase computed tomography (CT) shows a defect in the spleen that extends to the capsule (*arrow*). **(B)** Coronal, arterial phase CT shows some enhancement in the defect and a perisplenic hematoma (*arrow*). The laceration defect is > 3 cm, making this a grade 3 splenic injury. **(C)** Coronal, delayed phase CT shows some enhancement in the defect. No contrast extravasation is present next to the spleen (*arrow*). **(D)** Axial, delayed phase CT shows a small focus of contrast in the defect and fluid next to the spleen (*arrow*).

■ Differential Diagnosis

- **Splenic laceration:** Splenic laceration results from traumatic injury to the spleen and is graded based on its imaging features.
- *Splenic infarction:* Results from splenic ischemia.

■ Essential Facts

- Splenic laceration can be life threatening and requires prompt imaging.
- Splenic injury grading is done using the American Association for the Surgery of Trauma splenic injury grading scale based on laceration, hematoma, and vascular injury.
- Grade 1: subcapsular hematoma involving < 10% of surface area; capsular tear < 1 cm depth.
- Grade 2: subcapsular hematoma involving 10–50% of surface area; capsular tear 1–3 cm depth.
- Grade 3: Subcapsular, > 50% surface area of ruptured subcapsular or parenchymal hematoma; intraparenchymal hematoma > 10 cm; laceration > 3 cm parenchymal depth.

- Grade 4: Laceration involving segmental or hilar vessels producing major devascularization (> 25% of spleen).
- Grade 5: Completely shattered spleen with hilar devascularizing injury.

■ Other Imaging Findings

- Ultrasound can detect blood in the upper abdomen.
- Splenic lacerations appear as areas of mixed echogenicity.

✓ Pearls and ✗ Pitfalls

✓ Splenic lacerations require contrast for adequate grading.
✓ Reviewing both coronal and axial images makes grading more accurate.
✗ Active extravasation always indicates arterial vascular injury.
✗ Repeat imaging may be needed to evaluate for delayed splenic rupture.

Case 53

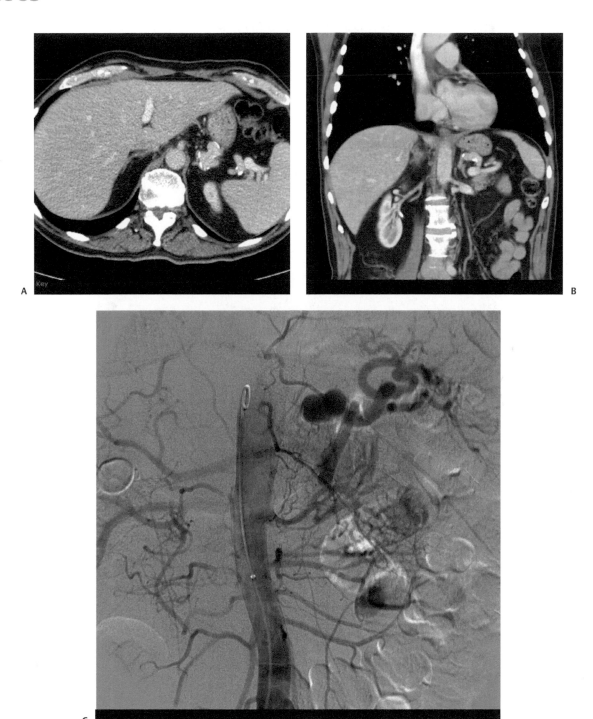

■ Clinical Presentation

A 79-year-old male undergoes computed tomography (CT) for abdominal pain.

■ **Imaging Findings**

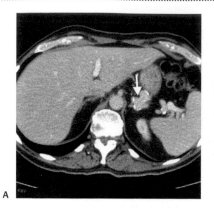
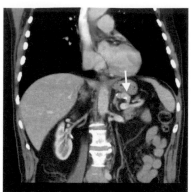

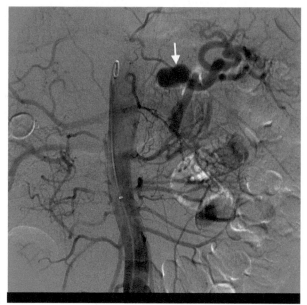

(A) Axial, contrast-enhanced CT shows a pseudoaneurysm from the splenic artery (*arrow*). **(B)** Coronal, contrast-enhanced CT shows the pseudoaneurysm from the splenic artery (*arrow*). **(C)** Catheter angiogram shows a nonthrombosed, ~3 cm aneurysm from the splenic artery (*arrow*).

■ **Differential Diagnosis**

- **Splenic artery pseudoaneurysm:** A pseudoaneurysm that arises from the splenic artery.
- *Tortuous splenic artery:* The splenic artery can be very tortuous and mimic an aneurysm.

■ **Essential Facts**

- Splenic artery pseudoaneurysms, although rare, are the most common visceral aneurysm.
- Causes include acute or chronic pancreatitis (21%), trauma, and pregnancy.
- More common in women (4:1) but higher rates of rupture in men.
- May be partially or fully thrombosed, and peripheral calcification is common.
- Splenic artery pseudoaneurysms range in size from < 1 to 17 cm (mean, 4.8 cm).

■ **Other Imaging Findings**

- Magnetic resonance imaging would detect the pseudoaneurysm on contrast-enhanced study; on a noncontrast study, a flow void may be detected.

✓ **Pearls and** ✗ **Pitfalls**

✓ Occurs in the distal third of the artery.
✓ The pseudoaneurysm may be peripherally calcified.
✗ A tortuous vessel can obscure a pseudoaneurysm.
✗ Measure the largest dimension of the vessel.

Case 54

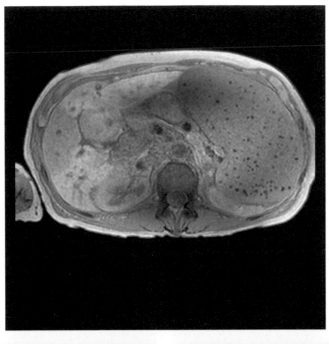

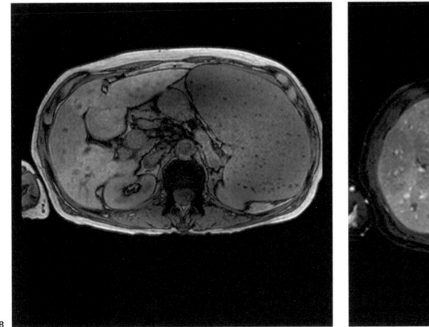

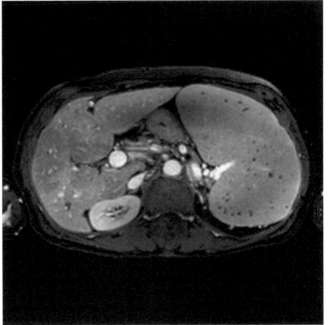

■ Clinical Presentation

A 60-year-old male with liver disease.

■ Imaging Findings

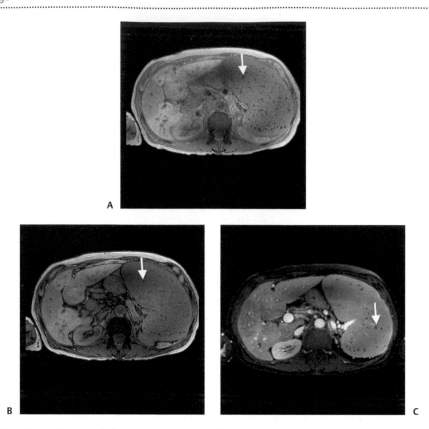

(A) In-phase T1-fast spoiled gradient echo (FSPGR) shows multiple tiny signal voids in an enlarged spleen (*arrow*). **(B)** Opposed-phase T1-FSPGR shows multiple tiny signal voids in an enlarged spleen (*arrow*). Note they are less evident than on the in-phase. **(C)** T1-postcontrast FSPGR shows no enhancement of the lesions (*arrow*).

■ Differential Diagnosis

- ***Gamna-Gandy bodies:*** Focal iron deposition due to microhemorrhages within the splenic parenchyma producing small siderotic nodules in patients with liver cirrhosis and portal hypertension.
- *Splenic granulomas:* Small calcifications that are the result of end-stage granulomatous infection.

■ Essential Facts

- Splenomegaly with hyperplasia of the cells of the reticulo-histiocytic system. Bleeding into the red pulpa with deposition of siderin adjacent to thickened collagen tissue forming so-called Gamna-Gandy bodies.
- Gamna-Gandy bodies contain fibrous tissue, hemosiderin, and calcium.
- They occur in patients with cirrhosis, portal or splenic vein thrombosis, hemolytic anemia, leukemia, lymphoma, acquired hemochromatosis, paroxysmal nocturnal hemoglobinuria, and patients receiving blood transfusions.
- Usually small (a few millimeters).
- They produce blooming on in-/opposed-phase magnetic resonance imaging (MRI).

■ Other Imaging Findings

- Noncontrast computed tomography (CT) may show faintly calcified nodules in the spleen.

✓ Pearls and ✗ Pitfalls

- ✓ Gamna-Gandy bodies may be used as a secondary sign of portal hypertension.
- ✓ Otherwise, they have little clinical value.
- ✗ They should not be confused for granulomata.
- ✗ They may not be detected by other modalities.

Case 55

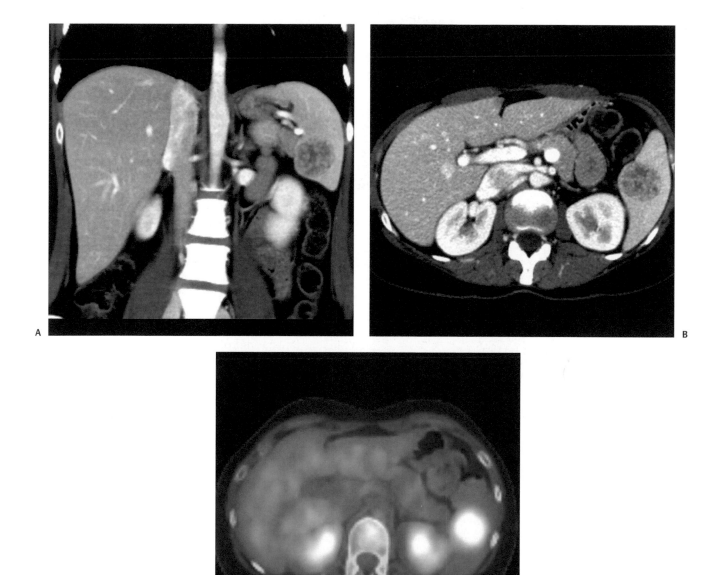

A

B

C

Clinical Presentation

A 40-year-old female with breast cancer undergoes staging computed tomography (CT) and F18–fluorodeoxyglucose (FDG) positron emission tomography (PET).

■ **Imaging Findings**

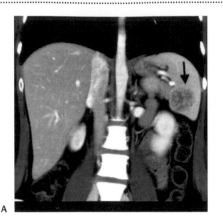 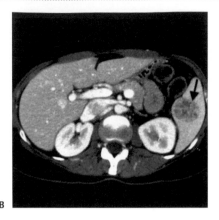 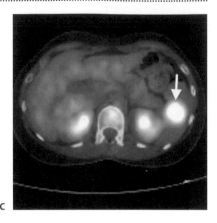

A   B   C

(A) Coronal, contrast-enhanced CT shows a well-circumscribed, hypoenhancing splenic mass in a normal-sized spleen (*arrow*). **(B)** Axial, contrast-enhanced CT shows a well-circumscribed, hypoenhancing splenic mass (*arrow*). **(C)** Axial F18-FDG PET shows the lesion to be markedly FDG avid (*arrow*).

■ **Differential Diagnosis**

• *Sclerosing angiomatoid nodular transformation (SANT):* Benign vascular lesion of the spleen with extensive sclerosis and unknown etiology.
• *Metastasis to the spleen:* Spleen forms a common site of metastasis for various malignancies.

■ **Essential Facts**

• SANT is a nonneoplastic vascular splenic lesion made up of dense fibrosis and angiomatoid nodules.
• Usually solitary.
• Well circumscribed on CT that hypoenhances relative to spleen.
• Tends to occur in females aged 30 to 60 years.

■ **Other Imaging Findings**

• SANT is hypoechoic on ultrasound. Hemorrhage can be detected on magnetic resonance imaging (MRI), and the lesion is one of the few splenic lesions that is T2-hypointense.

✓ **Pearls and ✗ Pitfalls**

✓ Well-circumscribed, solitary lesion.
✓ Lesions have old hemorrhage, dense fibrosis, and centripetal enhancement.
✗ Mimics can include solitary metastasis.
✗ FDG-PET can show avid uptake and can be mistaken for splenic disease in a patient undergoing staging for a malignancy.

Case 56

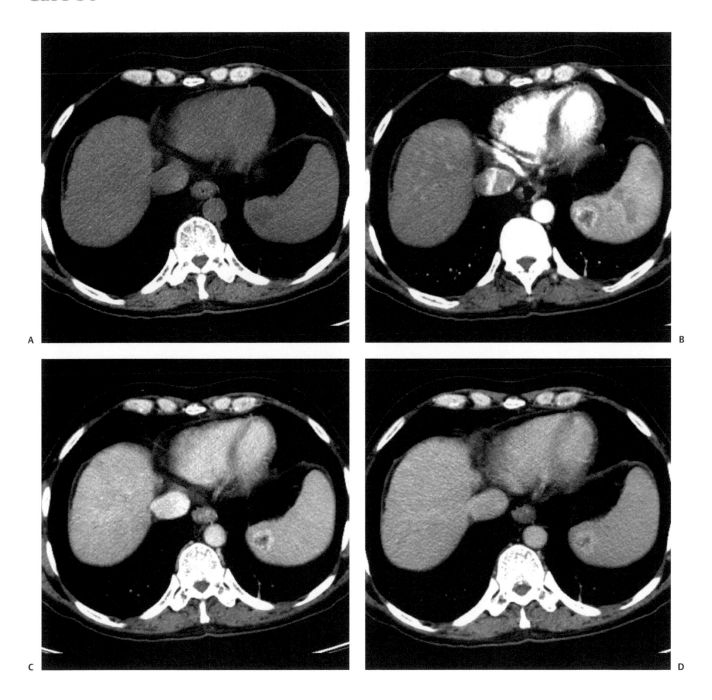

A

B

C

D

■ Clinical Presentation

A 68-year-old male with an incidental splenic lesion seen on a screening computed tomography (CT) performed for cirrhosis.

■ **Imaging Findings**

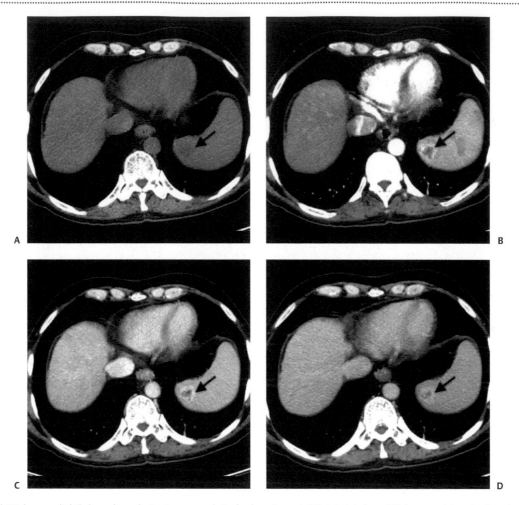

(A) Unenhanced CT shows a slightly hypodense lesion in a normal sized spleen (*arrow*). **(B)** Arterial phase CT shows peripheral enhancing rim of variable thickness (*arrow*). **(C)** Portal phase CT shows slight fill in of the lesion with contrast (*arrow*). **(D)** Delayed phase CT shows the lesion almost completely fills in with contrast and there is no washout (*arrow*).

■ **Differential Diagnosis**

- ***Splenic hemangioma:*** Rare, benign splenic vascular lesion that form by proliferation of vascular channels.
- *Littoral cell angioma:* Rare, benign vascular splenic lesion that is composed of littoral cells that line the splenic sinuses of the red pulp.

■ **Essential Facts**

- Splenic hemangiomas are rare, benign congenital vascular lesions of the spleen.
- Size can vary 0.5 to 7 cm; large splenic hemangiomas have been reported to rupture.
- Classic imaging findings are peripheral enhancement with focal areas of nodular enhancement and progressive centripetal enhancement on CT and magnetic resonance imaging.
- They arise from sinusoidal epithelium and most are the cavernous type.

■ **Other Imaging Findings**

- Splenic hemangiomas are typically T2-hyperintense and, unlike hepatic hemangiomas, tend to have a continuous rim of enhancement that has variable thickness and areas of nodular focal enhancement.

✓ **Pearls and** ✗ **Pitfalls**

- ✓ Lesions are usually well-defined and small.
- ✓ Lesions can have calcifications.
- ✗ Thrombosed or partially thrombosed lesions do not have the typical enhancement pattern.
- ✗ Biopsy carries an increased risk of bleeding compared with other splenic lesions.

Case 57

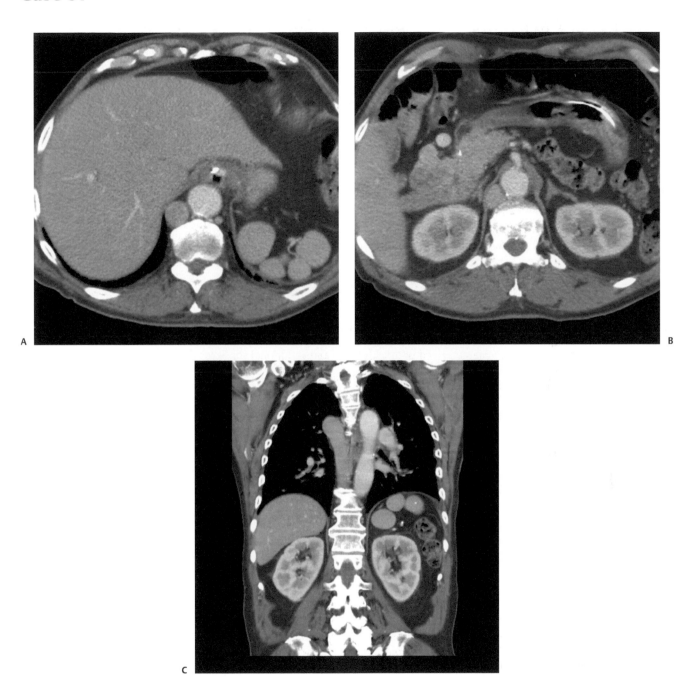

A

B

C

■ Clinical Presentation
....

A 50-year-old male with abdominal pain.

■ Imaging Findings

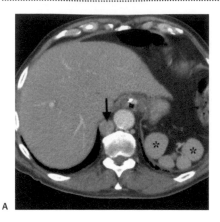 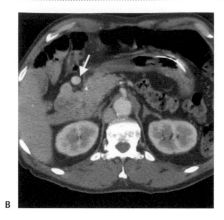 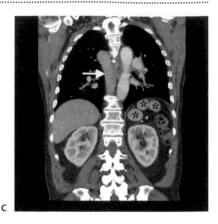

A   B   C

(A) Axial contrast-enhanced computed tomography (CT) shows multiple splenules, an absent inferior vena cava (IVC), and a distended azygous vein (*arrow, asterisks*). **(B)** Axial contrast-enhanced CT shows an absent IVC. Note that the portal vein (*arrow*) travels anterior to the duodenum. **(C)** Coronal contrast-enhanced CT shows the distended azygous vein and the polysplenia, and situs solitus (*arrow, asterisks*).

■ Differential Diagnosis

- ***Polysplenia with azygous continuation of the IVC:***
  Congenital heterotaxy syndrome characterized with polysplenia and absent suprarenal IVC. It is classically termed left isomerism or bilateral left-sidedness.

■ Essential Facts

- More common in females.
- Duplication of left-sided structures with bilateral bilobed lungs.
- Multiple spleens (2–16) always on the same side as the stomach.
- Supra renal segment of the IVC is absent.
- Drainage is via a large azygous vein.
- Associated with cardiac anomalies.
- Anomalies of the dorsal pancreas lead to a short pancreas.
- A preduodenal portal vein may be present.

■ Other Imaging Findings

- Chest radiography can show the dilated azygous vein and abdominal sonography can evaluate the polysplenia. There is duplication of left-sided structures with bilateral bilobed lungs, bilateral hyparterial bronchi, and bilateral pulmonary atria.

✓ Pearls and ✗ Pitfalls

- ✓ The interrupted IVC is a reliable finding in heterotaxy syndrome.
- ✓ The following structures should be evaluated: side of systemic and pulmonary atria, cardiac apex, aortic arch and descending aorta, the bronchial and lobar lung anatomy, the IVC, azygous vein, and the location of the stomach, liver, pancreas, portal vein, gallbladder, and splenic tissue.
- ✗ Intestinal malrotation can occur and viscera-atrial situs is variable.
- ✗ Anomalies of the dorsal pancreas lead to a short or truncated pancreas producing a short pancreatic duct.

Case 58

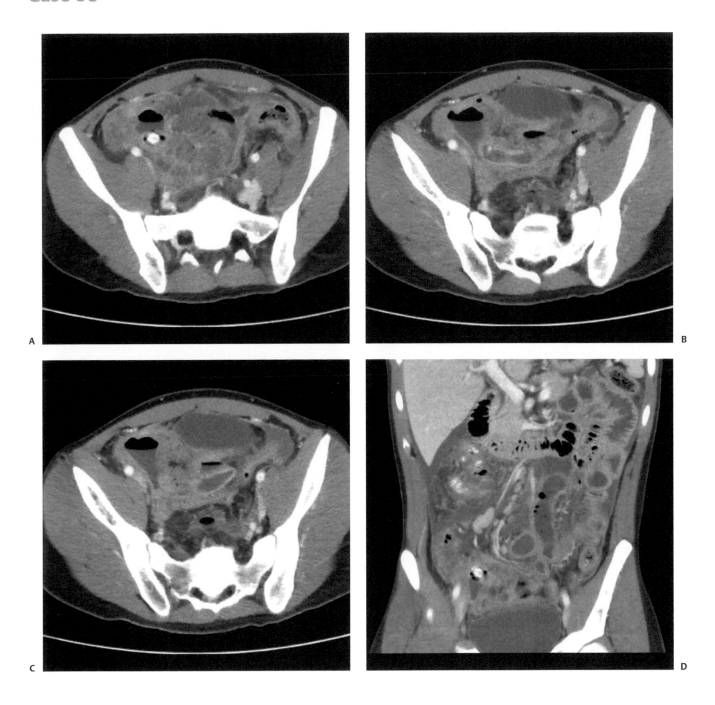

A

B

C

D

◼ Clinical Presentation

A 20-year-old male with abdominal pain and fever.

■ Imaging Findings

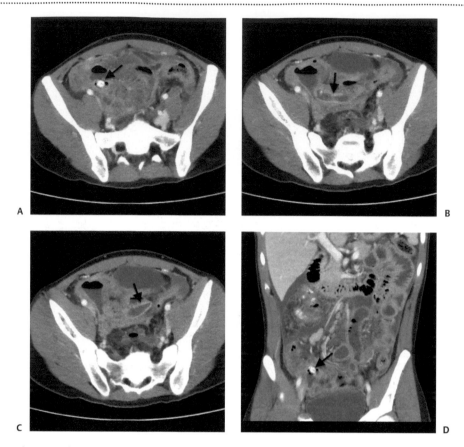

(A) Axial contrast-enhanced computed tomography (CT) shows thickened bowel segments and a focal calcification (appendicolith) in the right lower quadrant (*arrow*). **(B)** Axial contrast-enhanced CT shows a tubular enhancing structure in the right lower quadrant with a thick enhancing wall (*arrow*). **(C)** Axial contrast-enhanced CT shows that the enhancing structure in the right lower quadrant with a thick enhancing wall is blind ending (*arrow*). **(D)** Coronal contrast-enhanced CT shows multiple fluid pockets in the abdomen with enhancing walls and the appendicolith in the right lower quadrant (*arrow*). Note the dilated loops of bowel from an ileus.

■ Differential Diagnosis

- ***Acute appendicitis with perforation:*** Results from rupture of an inflamed appendix with associated abscess formation.
- *Meckel's diverticulum:* True intestinal diverticulum that can contain gastric or pancreatic tissue.

■ Essential Facts

- Imaging findings of acute appendicitis include appendiceal wall enhancement, periappendiceal fat stranding, intraluminal gas, appendicolith, ascites, ileus, and distention of the appendix.
- Findings of rupture may include appendiceal wall enhancement defect, extraluminal gas, extraluminal appendicolith, and abscess.

■ Other Imaging Findings

- Ultrasound can detect acute appendicitis in the appropriate patient but may not detect complications such as perforation indicated by abscess formation or extraluminal gas.
- Magnetic resonance imaging is used in pregnant patients in cases of suspected appendicitis.

✓ Pearls and ✗ Pitfalls

- ✓ The use of intravenous contrast is necessary to identify wall enhancement, wall defects, and abscess.
- ✓ The use of positive oral contrast helps in identifying interloop abscess.
- ✗ Perforated appendicitis can be missed because, at times, the appendix is not distinctly identified following rupture; in such cases, secondary signs should be used to infer a diagnosis.
- ✗ Pelvic inflammatory disease involving the right adnexa can mimic appendicitis as there is fat infiltration and, at times, serositis causing appendiceal wall enhancement.

Case 59

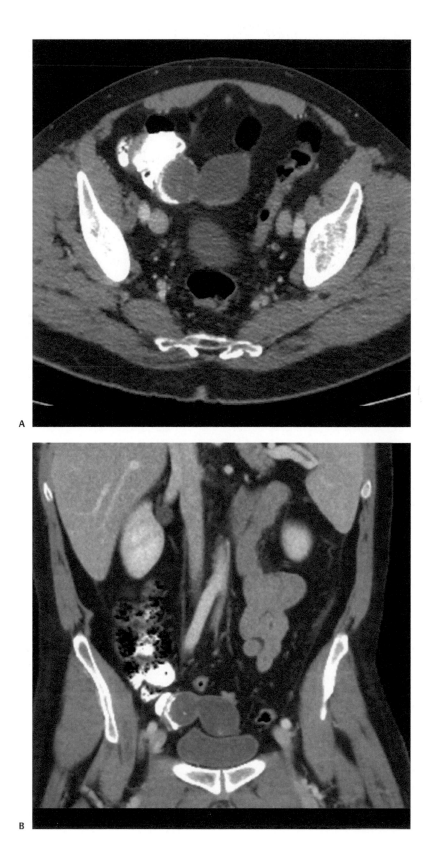

A

B

■ Clinical Presentation

A 59-year-old male with abdominal pain.

■ Imaging Findings

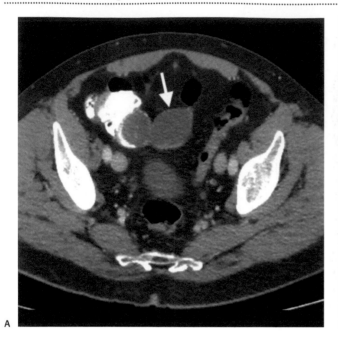 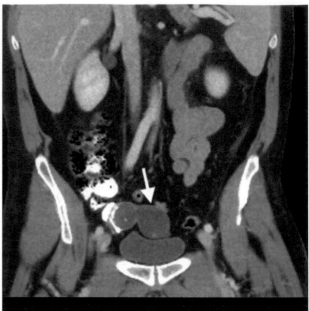

A   B

(A) Axial contrast-enhanced computed tomography (CT) shows a dilated lobular appendix filled with homogeneous low-attenuation material (*arrow*). The appendix does not fill with oral contrast. The appendiceal wall is thin and enhancing without surrounding inflammatory changes. (B) Coronal contrast-enhanced CT shows a dilated appendix that does not fill with oral contrast (*arrow*). Note the bulge into the base of the cecum.

■ Differential Diagnosis

- ***Appendiceal mucocele:*** Dilated, mucin-filled appendix with malignant potential.
- *Lymphoma of the appendix:* Involvement of the appendix by lymphoma that results in a thick-walled dilated appendix.

■ Essential Facts

- Mucocele of the appendix is a macroscopic descriptive term for a distended and mucin-filled appendix caused by several entities: simple mucous retention cyst, low-/high-grade appendiceal mucinous neoplasm, mucinous adenocarcinoma, obstruction of the appendix (e.g., caused by endometriosis), and inspissated mucous caused by cystic fibrosis.
- Appendiceal mucoceles usually dilate the appendix and have a thin, enhancing wall.
- Nodular enhancement, thick walls, soft tissue around the appendix, and ascites are signs that the tumor may have extended past the appendix.
- Peripheral wall calcifications can be present in appendiceal mucoceles.
- Treatment is a right hemicolectomy and nodal dissection as opposed to a simple appendectomy for acute appendicitis.

■ Other Imaging Findings

- Magnetic resonance imaging (MRI) will show a distended appendix, but the signal intensity may differ depending on the protein composition of the mucin.
- Ultrasound can show the dilated appendix and wall calcifications.

✓ Pearls and ✗ Pitfalls

- ✓ In 30–50% of cases, appendiceal tumors manifest clinically as acute appendicitis.
- ✓ Appendiceal epithelial neoplasms may present as pseudomyxoma peritonei.
- ✗ Mucoceles can become infected and demonstrate intraluminal gas or air-fluid levels, wall thickening, and surrounding fat stranding, mimicking acute appendicitis.
- ✗ Colonoscopy is not a good screening tool with a sensitivity of only 11% for appendiceal adenocarcinoma.

Case 60

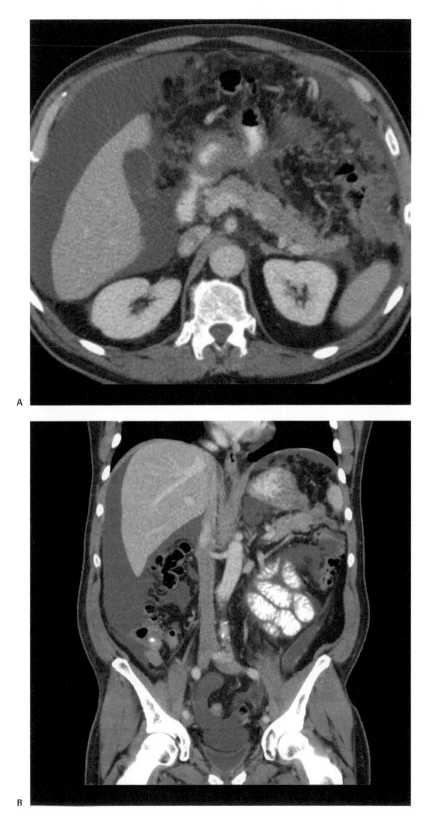

■ Clinical Presentation

A 74-year-old male with abdominal pain and bloating.

■ Imaging Findings

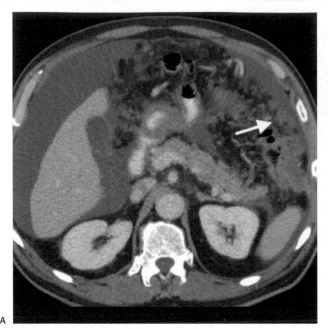 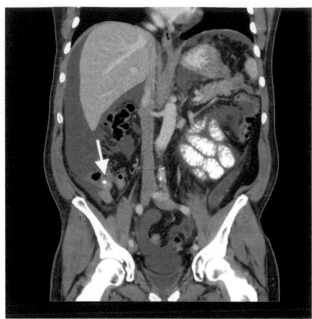

A   B

(A) Axial contrast-enhanced computed tomography (CT) shows nodularity of the omentum and upper abdominal ascites indicating carcinomatosis (*arrow*).
(B) Coronal contrast-enhanced CT shows a thickened appendix with a calcification at its base (*arrow*).

■ Differential Diagnosis

- ***Mucinous adenocarcinoma of the appendix:*** Mucinous neoplasm of the appendix that can cause peritoneal carcinomatosis and pseudomyxoma peritonei.
- *Carcinomatosis from unknown primary:* Carcinomatosis from many gastrointestinal and genitourinary malignancies can appear similar. The appendix is a frequent site of metastasis and can be thickened, mimicking a primary malignancy.

■ Essential Facts

- Mucinous adenocarcinoma can seed the peritoneum with mucin deposits and/or soft tissue deposits.
- The staging is surgical, based on the peritoneal cancer index.
- Treatment is surgical debulking and intra-abdominal chemotherapy.
- Recurrence is common.
- Histologically, signet ring morphology has the worst prognosis.
- Patients can present with multifocal bowel obstruction.

■ Other Imaging Findings

- Magnetic resonance imaging (MRI) is more sensitive than CT for peritoneal carcinomatosis and has a reported sensitivity of 84% for detection of small peritoneal implants compared with 54% for CT. Solid peritoneal and serosal tumors show restricted diffusion on diffusion-weighted imaging (DWI).
- Positron emission tomography (PET)/CT is typically not used in the setting of mucinous tumor as the cellular content is low, resulting in low fluorodeoxyglucose uptake and a sensitivity of only 35%.

✓ Pearls and ✗ Pitfalls

- ✓ CT underestimates the peritoneal carcinomatosis.
- ✓ Exams should be performed with oral and intravenous contrast.
- ✗ Pitfall areas include disease along the undersurface of the diaphragms, or near the spleen, lesser sac, and paracolic gutters.
- ✗ Appendiceal adenocarcinoma may mimic acute appendicitis by causing obstruction of the appendix, a thick appendiceal wall, and the lack of luminal contrast filling.

Case 61

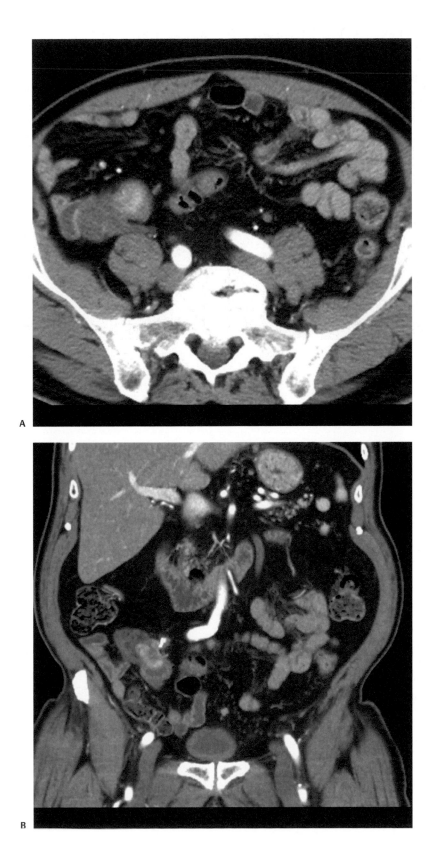

A

B

■ Clinical Presentation

A 75-year-old male with a history of hematuria undergoes computed tomography (CT).

■ **Imaging Findings**

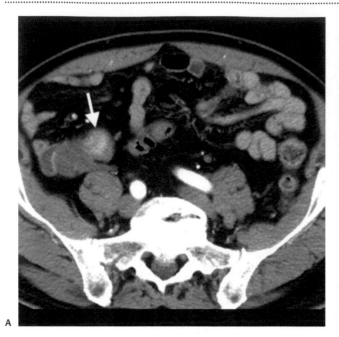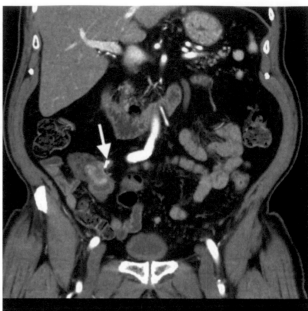

A   B

(A) Axial contrast-enhanced CT shows an enhancing mass in the ileocecal valve (*arrow*); the appendix is posterior and normal. **(B)** Coronal contrast-enhanced CT shows an enhancing mass in the ileocecal valve (*arrow*); note the calcification in the adjacent lymph node.

■ **Differential Diagnosis**

• ***Neuroendocrine tumor:*** Tumors from endocrine cells in the gastrointestinal tract that are derived from the neural crest, neuroectoderm, and endoderm. They can be functioning or nonfunctioning.
• *Small bowel gastrointestinal stromal tumor:* Rare malignant mesenchymal tumor of the small bowel.

■ **Essential Facts**

• Gastrointestinal neuroendocrine tumors involve the small intestine (30.8%), rectum (26.3%), colon (17.6%), pancreas (12.1%), stomach (8.9%), and appendix (5.7%).
• Histologically separated into well-differentiated endocrine tumors, well-differentiated endocrine carcinomas, and poorly differentiated endocrine carcinomas based on their location, histologic features, and biological behavior.
• Imaging features of neuroendocrine tumors can be variable from small, submucosal lesions to mucosal polypoid tumors.
• Neuroendocrine carcinomas can be polypoid or ulcerative and may metastasize.

■ **Other Imaging Findings**

• On magnetic resonance imaging, neuroendocrine tumors are isointense to muscle on T1-weighted imaging and either hyperintense or isointense to muscle on T2-weighted imaging.
• Lesions show enhancement after the administration of an intravenous contrast agent.

✓ **Pearls and** ✗ **Pitfalls**

✓ Small mucosal lesions may not be evident; in such cases, the calcified nodes or mesenteric masses may indicate the presence of a neuroendocrine tumor.
✓ The primary tumor can be smaller than the metastatic deposits.
✗ Portal venous phase CT may miss mucosal lesions as they tend to be hypervascular.
✗ Appendiceal neuroendocrine tumors may present as appendicitis.

Case 62

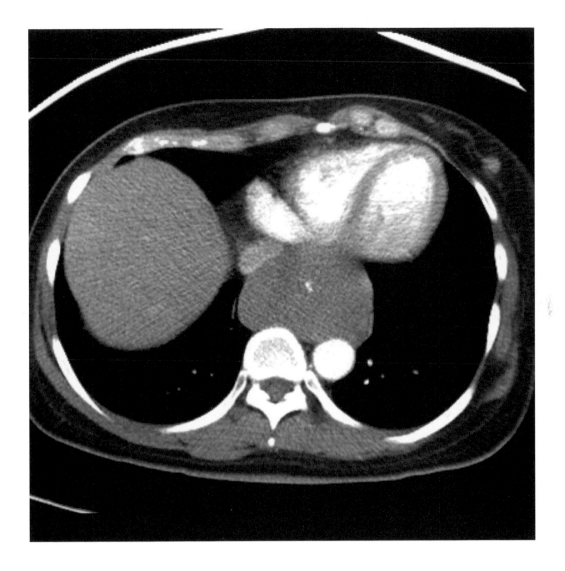

■ **Clinical Presentation**

A 40-year-old male with dysphagia.

■ **Imaging Findings**

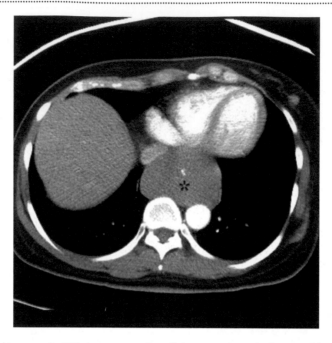

(A) Axial contrast-enhanced computed tomography (CT) shows a smooth, well-demarcated mass in the area of the distal esophagus with a central calcification (*asterisk*). The lesion is deformed by the contour of the aorta.

■ **Differential Diagnosis**

- ***Esophageal leiomyoma:*** Rare benign mesenchymal smooth muscle tumor of the esophagus with spindle cells.
- *Esophageal gastrointestinal stromal tumor:* Rare malignant mesenchymal tumor of the esophagus with spindle cell and epithelioid cell types.

■ **Essential Facts**

- Esophageal leiomyomas can be small or large; large lesions cause symptomatic mass effect.
- They can displace or compress the esophagus.
- They exhibit midlevel enhancement on CT.
- The presence of calcifications is most specific for the diagnosis.
- Most esophageal leiomyomas arise from the muscularis propria; 80% are intramural and 7% are extraesophageal.
- Most arise in the mid- to distal third of the esophagus, where there is an increased ratio of smooth muscle to striated muscle in the esophageal wall.
- They are associated with other benign esophageal conditions such as achalasia, esophageal diverticulum, and gastroesophageal reflux. The most commonly associated condition is hiatal hernia, which is found in 4.5 to 23% of patients with leiomyoma.

■ **Other Imaging Findings**

- On barium upper gastrointestinal tract radiography, esophageal leiomyomas form a smooth submucosal mass with narrowing of the lumen with obtuse margins.

✓ **Pearls and ✗ Pitfalls**

✓ Oral contrast in the esophagus and intravenous contrast help evaluate the lesion.
✓ Presence of calcifications is helpful in diagnosing the entity.
✗ Necrosis, invasion, and esophageal obstruction are suggestive of malignant degeneration.
✗ Its location can mimic esophageal duplication cysts and pericardial cysts.

Case 63

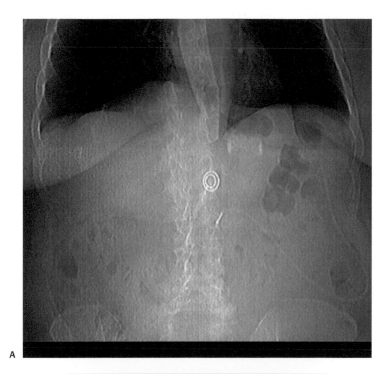

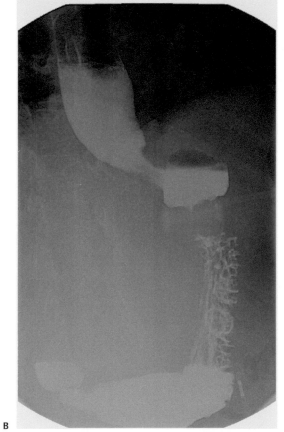

A 55-year-old female with abdominal pain.

■ **Imaging Findings**

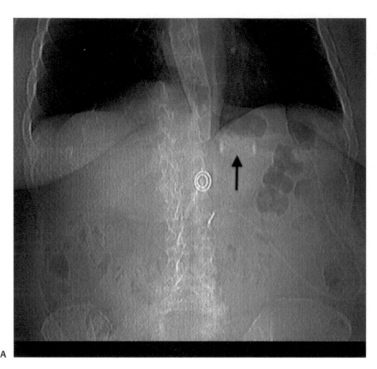
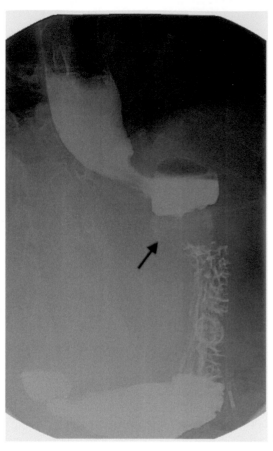

(A) Computed tomography (CT) scout image shows a gastric band in a near horizontal position (*arrow*); note the gastric gas bubble above the band. The Phi angle is about 85 degrees. (B) Single contrast barium study shows that the gastric band has slipped and now constricts the proximal gastric body (*arrow*). There is inferior displacement of the band and an air-fluid level above the band.

■ **Differential Diagnosis**

• **Slipped gastric band:** Gastric band slippage is one of the possible complications of the laparoscopic gastric band.

■ **Essential Facts**

• Gastric band slippage occurs in about 10% of cases.
• The Phi angle is the angle formed between the perpendicular line of the spinous processes and the line through the band.
• A normal Phi angle is 4 to 58 degrees. A Phi angle > 58 degrees is 91–95% sensitive and 52–62% specific for gastric band slippage.
• Displacement of the superolateral band margin by more than 2.4 cm from the diaphragm is the most sensitive and specific sign.
• The "O-Sign" is formed with abnormal positioning of the band so its visible enface; the sign is very specific.
• A tight gastric band will produce distention of the pouch > 4 cm.
• Possible complications of perforation and gastric erosion are best evaluated by CT.

■ **Other Imaging Findings**

• Anteroposterior radiographs of the abdomen are the best option for evaluation of the Phi angle. In cases of perforation or erosion, there can be fluid around the stomach, abscess pockets, or free gas in the abdomen.

✓ **Pearls and ✗ Pitfalls**

✓ The CT scout film or a radiograph is most helpful in determining the angle of the gastric band.
✓ Look for signs of gastric obstruction such as a dilated gastric pouch or esophagus.
✗ The slipped band can cause erosion or perforation of the stomach, which can be missed on radiographs or even barium exams.
✗ Malfunction, kinking, or discontinuity of the tubing can cause malfunction of the band.

Case 64

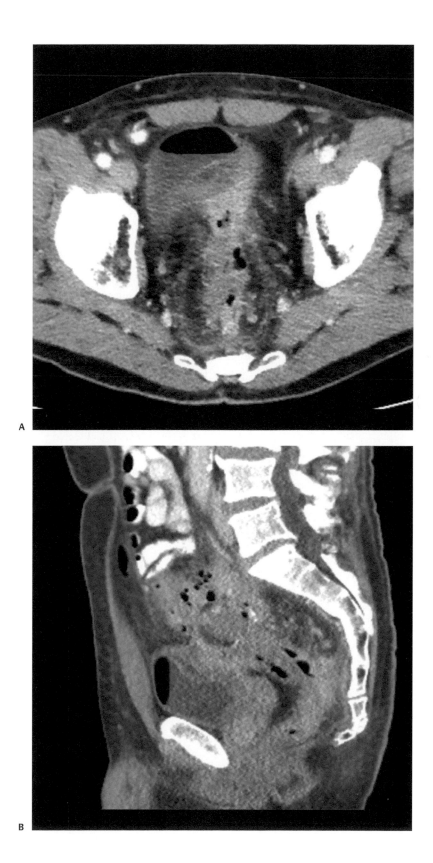

A

B

■ Clinical Presentation

A 60-year-old male with abdominal pain and pneumaturia.

■ **Imaging Findings**

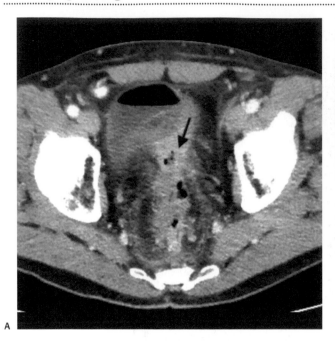 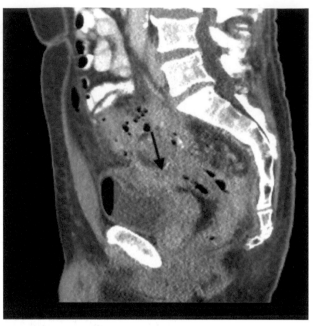

(A) Axial contrast-enhanced computed tomography (CT) shows gas in the lumen of the bladder, sigmoid colonic wall thickening, inflammation, and a soft tissue tract from the colon to the bladder (*arrow*). (B) Sagittal contrast-enhanced CT shows extensive diverticular disease, inflammation, and fat stranding (*arrow*).

■ **Differential Diagnosis**

- ***Colonic diverticulitis with colovesical fistula:***
  Diverticular inflammation resulting in a fistula between the colon and the urinary bladder.
- *Colonic adenocarcinoma with colovesical fistula:*
  Carcinoma of the colon resulting in a fistula between the colon and the urinary bladder.
- *Fistulizing Crohn's disease:* Transmural inflammatory disease that results in fistulae, strictures, and abscess.

■ **Essential Facts**

- Most common cause of colovesical fistula is diverticulitis, which accounts for ~65 to 79% of cases.
- Pneumaturia, fecaluria, and suprapubic pain are the most common presenting signs and symptoms.
- The presence of gas in the urinary bladder is a specific sign of a fistula.
- In some cases, a direct connection may be visible.
- CT has a reported sensitivity of 61%.

■ **Other Imaging Findings**

- Magnetic resonance imaging can show the fistulous connection and in some cases is as sensitive as CT.

✓ **Pearls and ✗ Pitfalls**

- ✓ Evaluation of the colon by colonoscopy is needed to exclude malignancy.
- ✓ Rectal contrast that enters the bladder or CT cystogram are additional tests to improve accuracy.
- ✗ The absence of a visible tract does not exclude a fistula.
- ✗ Gas in the urinary bladder may be from recent manipulation and not necessarily from a fistula. Clinical history is needed.

Case 65

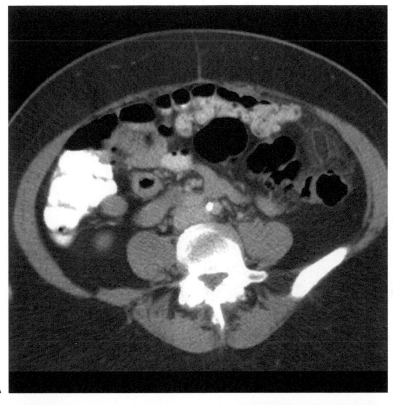

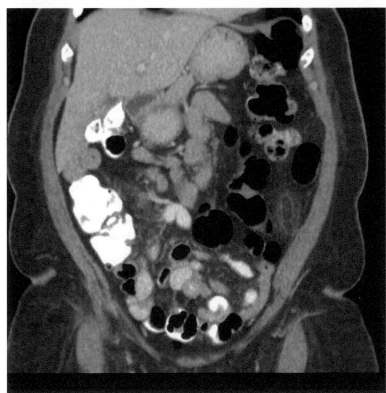

■ Clinical Presentation

A 55-year-old female with left lower quadrant abdominal pain.

■ Imaging Findings

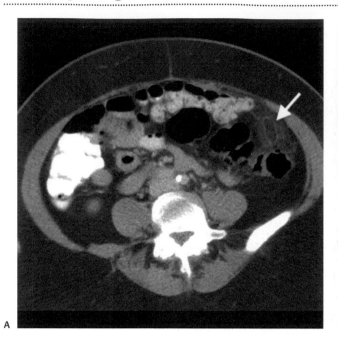 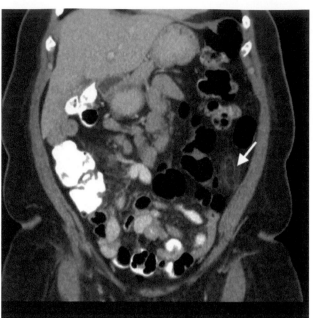

A   B

(A) Axial contrast-enhanced computed tomography (CT) shows an ovoid fat density mass surrounded by a hyperattenuating ring (*arrow*). (B) Coronal contrast-enhanced CT shows a thin, hyperattenuating ring surrounding ovoid fatty mass (*arrow*).

■ Differential Diagnosis

- ***Epiploic appendagitis:*** Benign, self-limiting inflammatory process of the epiploic appendages.
- *Acute diverticulitis:* Acute inflammation of colonic diverticula.

■ Essential Facts

- Epiploic appendagitis results from torsion of epiploic appendages and commonly occurs in the sigmoid colon; the second most common site is the cecum.
- It is imaged as a fatty mass with a hyperattenuating ring.
- Rarely, epiploic appendagitis can have surrounding inflammation and a central hyperattenuating focus from venous thrombosis.
- Self-limiting entity.

■ Other Imaging Findings

- Magnetic resonance imaging can show a fat attenuation center with a low attenuation rim on T1-weighted imaging. The rim enhances on postcontrast imaging.

✓ Pearls and ✗ Pitfalls

- ✓ The presence of a fatty mass abutting the colon should raise suspicion for epiploic appendagitis.
- ✓ Omental infarcts tend to be larger.
- ✗ Epiploic appendagitis may be confused with acute diverticulitis if it occurs on the left.
- ✗ Epiploic appendagitis can be confused with acute appendicitis if it occurs about the cecum.

Case 66

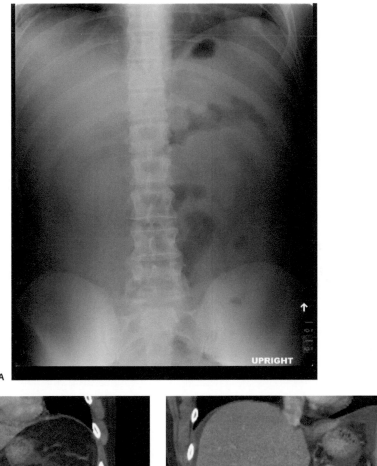

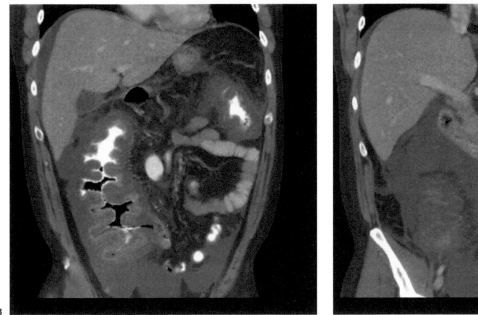

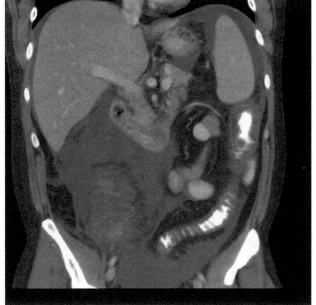

■ Clinical Presentation

A 40-year-old male with abdominal pain, bloody stool, and fever.

■ Imaging Findings

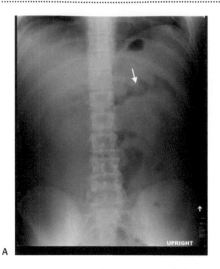
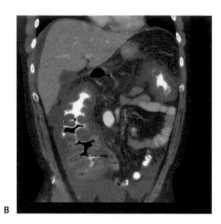
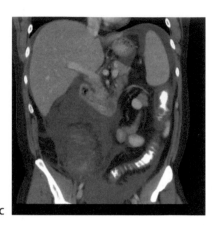

A   B   C

(A) Anteroposterior abdominal radiograph shows colonic haustral thickening and a nonobstructive bowel gas pattern (*arrow*). **(B, C)** Coronal contrast-enhanced computed tomography shows a pancolitis with severe colonic wall thickening and nodularity, pericolonic stranding/edema, and ascites. Note the trapped oral contrast between nodular thickened folds producing the "accordion sign."

■ Differential Diagnosis

- **Pseudomembranous colitis:** Infectious colitis from the gram-positive, anaerobic pathogen *Clostridium difficile.*
- *Inflammatory bowel disease:* Autoimmune or idiopathic inflammation of the bowel.
- *Low protein state:* Low albumin states cause third spacing and diffuse bowel wall thickening.

■ Essential Facts

- Pseudomembranous colitis is infectious colitis caused by gram-positive, anaerobic *Clostridium difficile.*
- There is severe colonic wall thickening (5 to 25 mm), the most accurate sign.
- Pericolonic fat infiltration.
- Ascites.
- Colonic wall nodularity.

■ Other Imaging Findings

- Magnetic resonance imaging shows diffuse colonic wall thickening with increased T2 signal in the edematous colon.

✓ Pearls and ✗ Pitfalls

- ✓ Rectal involvement was the most common site (90–95%).
- ✓ Dilation of the colon and shock can indicate toxic megacolon, a possible life-threatening complication of infectious colitis.
- ✗ Bowel perforation may be difficult to detect in the presence of ascites without the presence of free gas.
- ✗ The entire colon may not be involved. In ~5% of cases, only the right and transverse colon are involved.

Case 67

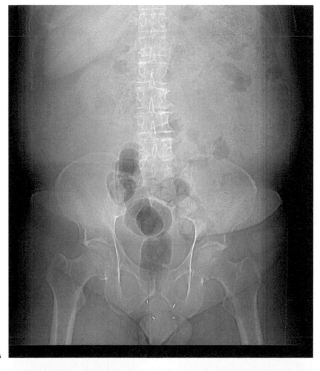

A

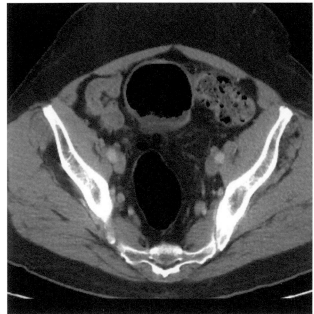

B

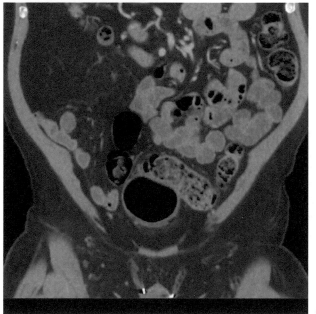

C

■ Clinical Presentation

A 69-year-old male with anemia and intermittent abdominal pain.

■ **Imaging Findings**

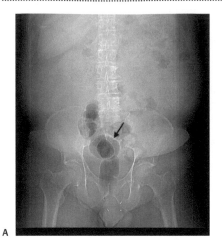
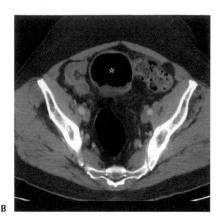
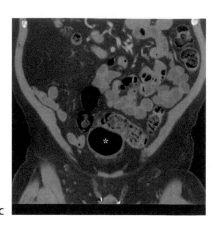

(A) Computed tomography (CT) scout shows a focal, rounded pocket of gas that projects over the sigmoid colon (*arrow*). **(B)** Axial CT shows a gas-filled pocket next to the sigmoid colon with a wall (*asterisk*). **(C)** Coronal CT shows a gas-filled pocket adjacent to the colon with some surrounding infiltration of the fat (*asterisk*).

■ **Differential Diagnosis**

- *Giant colonic diverticulum:* Rare complication of diverticular disease resulting in a large diverticulum.
- *Abdominal abscess:* Infected collection in the abdomen that can contain gas and fluid.
- *Large-bowel volvulus:* Twisting of the large bowel with resultant dilation.

■ **Essential Facts**

- Giant colonic diverticulum is defined as a diverticulum > 4 cm.
- They are most commonly associated with the sigmoid colon (90%), and abdominal pain is the most common complaint (70%). Intermittent obstruction can cause clinical signs of infection.
- Smooth-walled, gas-filled structure in contact with the colon. May be partially or fully filled with fluid.
- There are three types: Type 1 diverticula (22%) represents a pseudodiverticula with remnants of muscularis mucosa and true muscularis; Type 2 (65%) is secondary to subserosal perforation with a walled-off abscess that gradually increases in size; Type 3 (13%) represents a true diverticulum that contains all four bowel layers and is most likely to have a congenital origin.
- Treatment is surgical with en bloc resection and anastomosis.

■ **Other Imaging Findings**

- Non-filling of the diverticulum with contrast may be due to a narrowed or obstructed ostium.

✓ **Pearls and ✗ Pitfalls**

✓ CT scout radiograph can help identify the diverticulum.
✓ Colonoscopy is rarely performed as there is a risk of perforation.
✗ May mimic a pericolonic abscess caused by perforation.
✗ Barium enema opacifies the diverticulum in ~60% of cases even though a communication may not be demonstrated.

Case 68

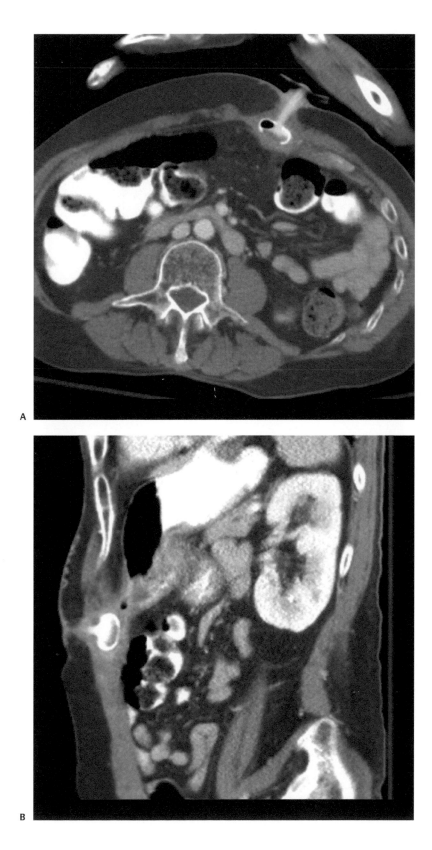

A

B

■ Clinical Presentation

A 60-year-old female with a malfunctioning gastrostomy tube.

■ **Imaging Findings**

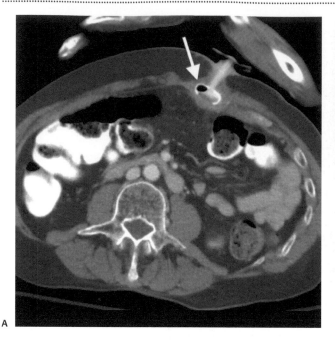
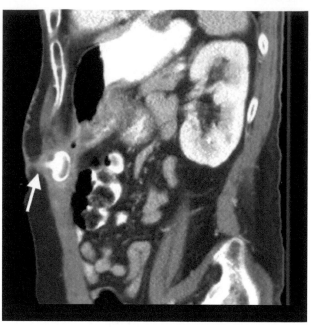

A   B

(A) Axial contrast-enhanced computed tomography (CT) shows the bumper of the gastrostomy tube retracted and adherent to the abdominal muscles (*arrow*). Note the soft tissue thickening around the bumper. **(B)** Sagittal contrast-enhanced CT shows the bumper buried in the wall of the abdomen with surrounding soft tissue thickening (*arrow*).

■ **Differential Diagnosis**

• **Buried bumper syndrome:** The internal bumper migrates alongside the stoma tract out of the stomach and is lodged in the soft tissues.

■ **Other Imaging Findings**

• Contrast instilled via the tube can show a fistulous connection with the stomach and can opacify the stomach lumen.

■ **Essential Facts**

• More prone with a rigid or semirigid internal fixation device and tight external fixator.
• Occurs in ~1% of percutaneous gastrostomy tubes.
• Leakage of contents is an early symptom.
• There is a fistula from the buried bolster to the stomach.
• A fixed bumper and occlusion are accurate signs of a severe form of the process.
• The distance from the external fixator and skin should be 10 mm.
• Treatment in advanced cases is endoscopic removal.

✓ **Pearls and ✗ Pitfalls**

✓ May be associated with an abscess.
✓ Use water-soluble contrast to interrogate the device.
✗ Blockage of the catheter is a late finding.
✗ Lower grades of buried bumper may be difficult to diagnose as it may be partly mobile and patent.

Case 69

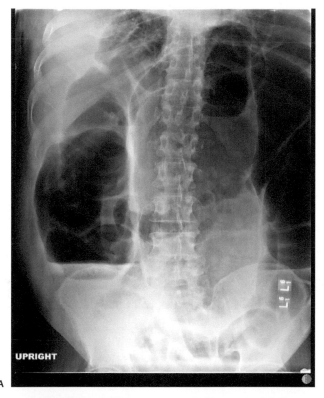

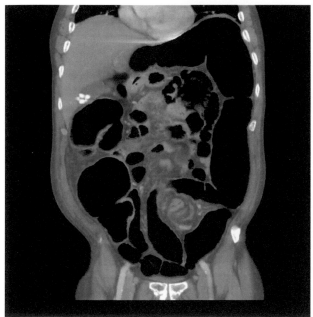

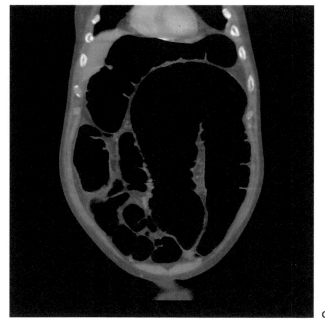

■ Clinical Presentation

A 70-year-old male with abdominal pain and inability to pass flatus.

■ **Imaging Findings**

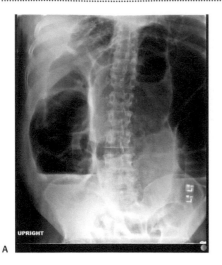
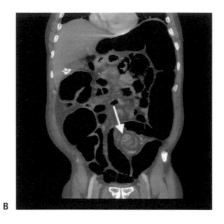
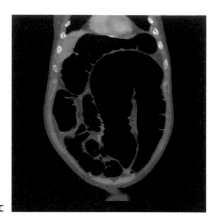

(A) Radiograph of the abdomen shows a distended colon shaped like a coffee bean with air-fluid levels. Note the three lines pointing toward the pelvis: the Frimann-Dahl sign. **(B)** Coronal computed tomography (CT) shows a twisting of the mesentery about the sigmoid colon with a classic "whirl" appearance (*arrow*). **(C)** Coronal CT shows the dilated loop of sigmoid colon.

■ **Differential Diagnosis**

- *Sigmoid volvulus:* Twisting of the sigmoid colon around its mesentery: the sigmoid mesocolon.
- *Distal colonic obstruction:* Distal colonic obstruction can mimic a sigmoid volvulus when the colon undergoes significant distention.

■ **Essential Facts**

- Sigmoid volvulus accounts for ~60% of colonic volvulus.
- Poor enhancement, pneumatosis, or wall thickening suggests ischemia.
- High density in the colon wall suggests hemorrhagic necrosis.

■ **Other Imaging Findings**

- Rectal barium contrast shows the narrowing of the lumen at the site of obstruction creating a bird-beak sign.

✓ **Pearls and** ✗ **Pitfalls**

- ✓ The lines of the twisted colonic segment point to the site of obstruction.
- ✓ Identifying the whirl of the vessels in the mesentery on CT helps confirm the diagnosis.
- ✗ Very distended and tortuous colon in patients with chronic colonic dilatation can impede diagnosis.
- ✗ Ischemia may be missed on plain radiography.

Case 70

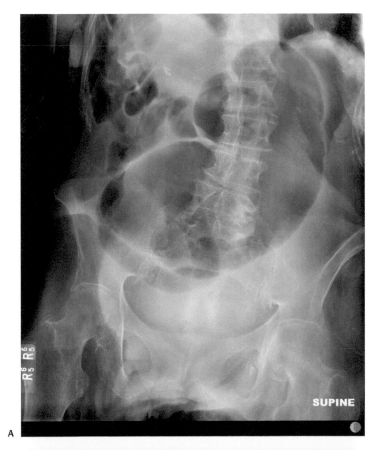

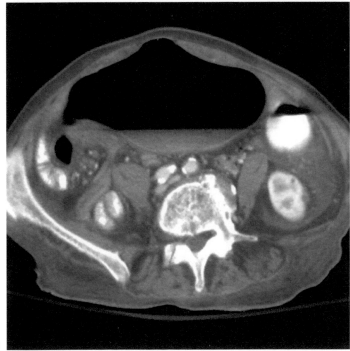

■ **Clinical Presentation**

A 90-year-old female with abdominal pain and failure to pass flatus.

■ Imaging Findings

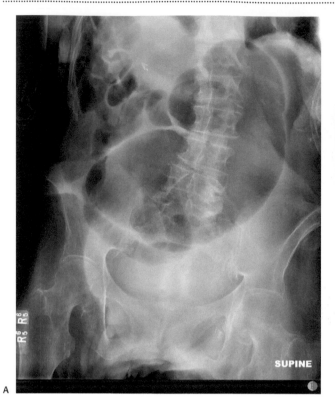

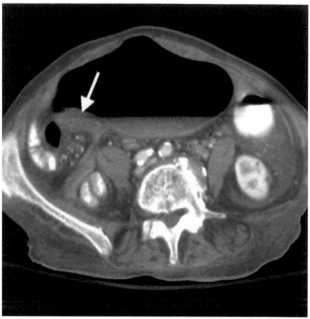

(A) Radiograph shows distended loop in the left upper abdomen shaped like a coffee bean. The presence of a haustral crease indicates its colonic origin. **(B)** Axial contrast-enhanced computed tomography (CT) shows the distended cecum; note the compressed colon sandwiched between loops of small bowel (*arrow*).

■ Differential Diagnosis

- ***Cecal volvulus:*** Torsion of the cecum around its mesentery.
- *Cecal obstruction:* Cecal obstruction from other causes leading to colonic distention.

■ Essential Facts

- Cecal volvulus accounts for ~40% of colonic volvulus.
- Cecal volvulus results in a closed loop obstruction of the cecum.
- The whirl sign is present in the right lower quadrant.
- There are three reported types: the bascule type, where the cecum is redundant and is simply anteriorly upturned; the loop type (most common), where the cecum is upturned and twisted around the axis of the colon; and the axial type, where there is a simple twist of the cecum around the axis of the colon without displacement.
- In the loop type, the cecum is located in the upper abdomen.
- CT scan can diagnose cecal volvulus with almost 100% sensitivity and > 90% specificity.

■ Other Imaging Findings

- On barium enema, the contrast column fills the colon and sharply tapers but may not fill the cecum depending on the extent of volvulus.

✓ Pearls and ✗ Pitfalls

- ✓ Evaluate for signs of ischemia such as bowel thickening, perforation, pneumatosis intestinalis, and ascites.
- ✓ The colon past the cecum is often decompressed, supporting the diagnosis.
- ✗ The cecal bascule can mimic a volvulus as it is distended.
- ✗ Barium enema should not be performed in ill patients, patients with suspected perforation, or cases of bowel gangrene.

Case 71

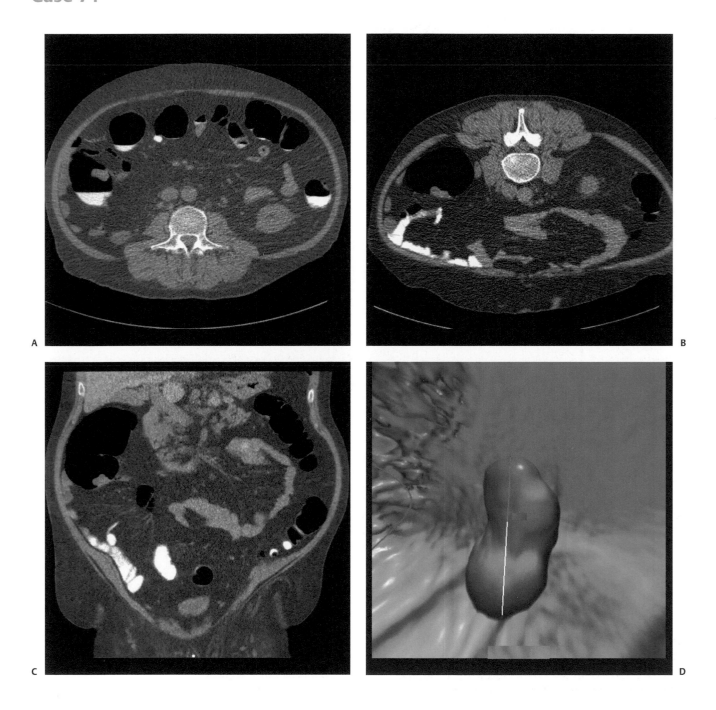

■ Clinical Presentation

A 65-year-old male undergoes computed tomography (CT) colonography for screening for colon cancer.

- ■ **Imaging Findings**

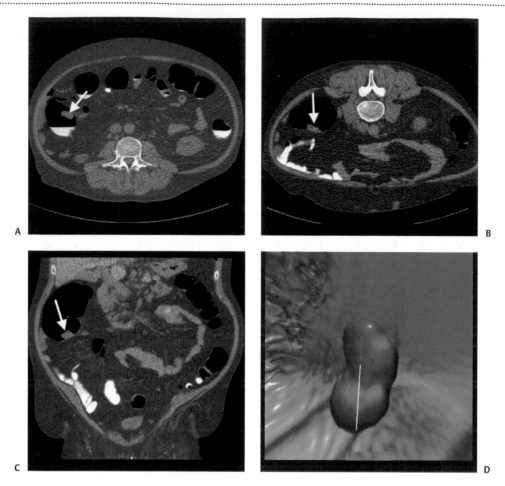

(A) Supine CT colonography shows a pedunculated polyp in the region of the ascending colon (*arrow*). No contrast coating is present on the polyp. **(B)** Prone CT colonography shows the polypoid mass has moved, and now lies flat against the colon wall (*arrow*). **(C)** Coronal CT colonography shows the polyp arising from the colon wall (*arrow*). **(D)** Endoluminal view of the colon shows the polypoid mass.

- ■ **Differential Diagnosis**

- **Tubulovillous adenoma:** Type of colonic polyp with tubular and villous elements.
- *Serrated adenoma:* Polyp with serrated architecture throughout the full length of the glands.
- *Tubular adenoma:* Small, pedunculated polyp composed of small rounded or tubular cells.
- *Villous adenoma:* Large, sessile polyp covered by slender villi.

- ■ **Essential Facts**

- When performing CT colonography, proper colonic preparation is needed for accurate interpretation.
- Oral contrast is used for tagging.
- Proper colonic insufflation is critical.
- Interpretation should include a primary two-dimensional read and endoluminal views.
- Lesion size, segmental location, and morphology (sessile, pedunculated, flat mass) should be documented.

- ■ **Other Imaging Findings**

- Double-contrast barium enema can be used in certain cases but has significant shortcomings, including a lower sensitivity than CT colonography (between 39% and 56%).

- ✓ **Pearls and** ✗ **Pitfalls**

- ✓ Proper patient preparation, cleansing, and tagging are important components of CT colonography.
- ✓ Colonic distention with carbon dioxide is the preferred method to distend the colon.
- ✗ Flat lesions can be difficult to detect.
- ✗ Lesions in and around the ileocecal valve or around the sigmoid colon in the setting of chronic diverticulosis with thickened folds can be challenging.

Case 72

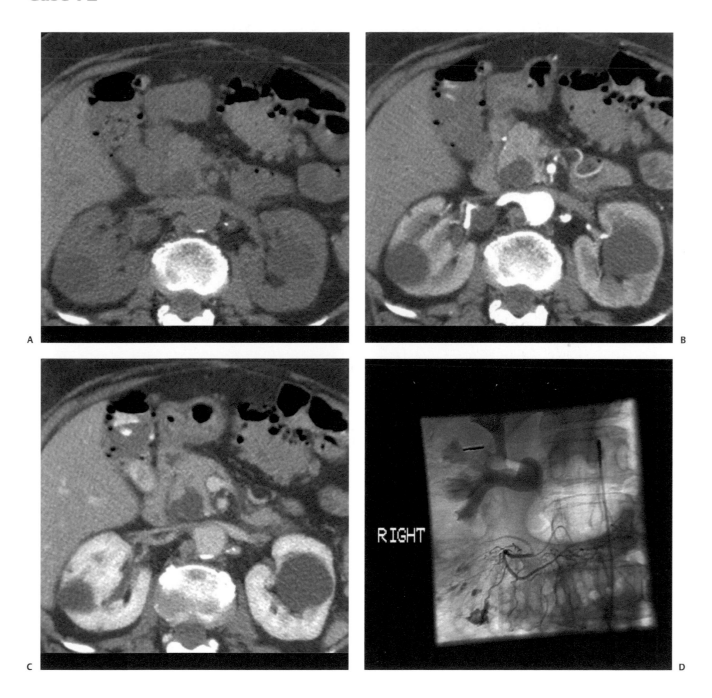

A

B

C

D

■ Clinical Presentation

An inpatient with profuse lower gastrointestinal (GI) bleeding.

■ Imaging Findings

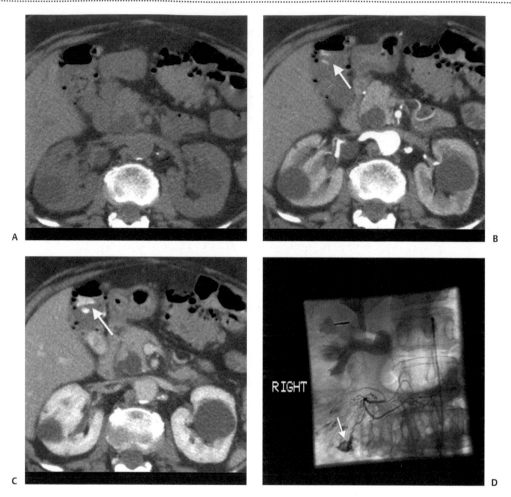

(A) Axial noncontrast computed tomography (CT) shows extensive colonic diverticulosis. **(B)** Axial arterial phase CT shows focal contrast extravasation in the colon (*arrow*). **(C)** Axial venous phase CT shows progressive contrast extravasation in the colon lumen (*arrow*). **(D)** Mesenteric angiogram shows brisk bleeding from the colon corresponding to the findings on CT (*arrow*).

■ Differential Diagnosis

• **Colonic bleed:** Arterial or venous bleeding from the colon.

■ Essential Facts

• The most common causes of colonic bleeding are diverticular bleeding (30%), hemorrhoids (14%), ischemia (12%), and inflammatory bowel disease (9%).
• Triple-phase CT angiography (CTA) with noncontrast, arterial phase and portal venous phase are performed.
• Oral contrast is not administered as neutral oral contrast may diminish sensitivity and delay the study.
• Contrast in a colonic bleed can appear as jet-like, swirled, circular/ellipsoid, pooled, or cloud-shaped.

■ Other Imaging Findings

• Technetium-99m scintigraphy can be performed with a sulfur colloid– or red blood cell–based radiopharmaceutical and is very sensitive for the detection of bleeds. However, it lacks anatomical information.

✓ Pearls and ✗ Pitfalls

✓ Perform the triple-phase CT immediately after the bleed. Bleeds may stop or be intermittent and result in a negative study.
✓ Do not administer oral contrast as this practice will delay the exam, limit interpretation, and reduce accuracy.
✗ Mucosal enhancement from collapsed bowel segments can mimic a bleed.
✗ High-attenuation fecal contents in diverticula limit the detection.

Case 73

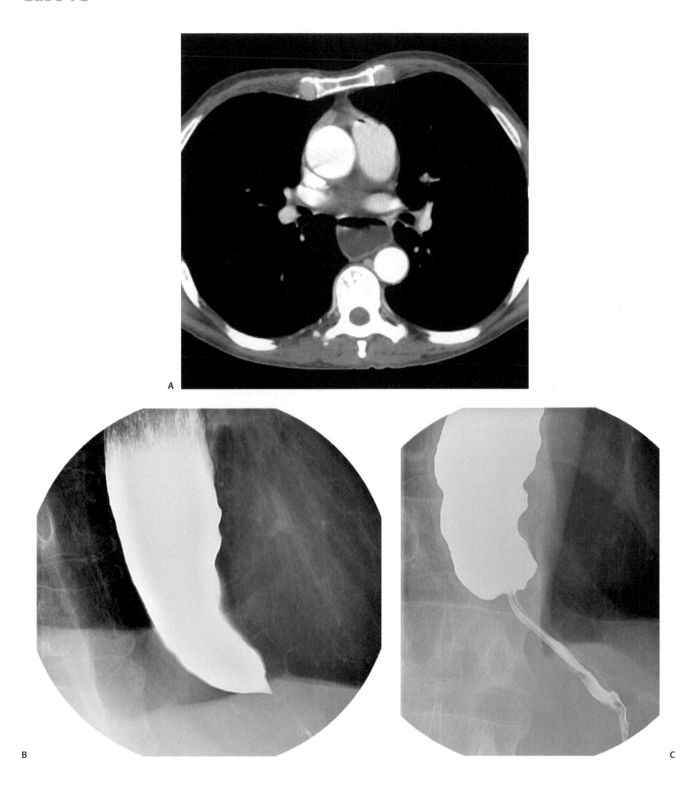

■ Clinical Presentation

A 70-year-old male complains of dysphagia to both solids and liquids accompanied by regurgitation and chest pain.

■ **Imaging Findings**

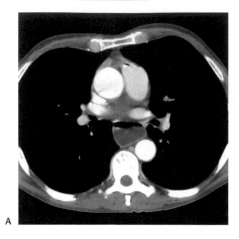 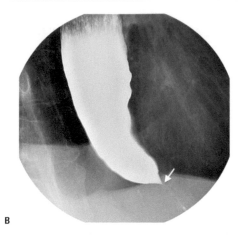 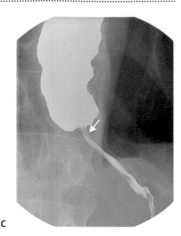

A   B   C

(A) Axial computed tomography shows a distended, fluid-filled esophagus with a thin wall. **(B)** Barium esophagogram shows a distended esophagus that tapers (*arrow*). **(C)** Barium esophagogram shows the persistent smooth stricture involving the distal esophagus (*arrow*). Note the central lucency surrounded by barium on both sides.

■ **Differential Diagnosis**

- ***Primary achalasia of the esophagus:*** Primary disorder of esophageal motility.
- *Pseudoachalasia (secondary achalasia):* Dilatation of the esophagus from other causes such as infection, malignancy, or other obstructing mass.

■ **Essential Facts**

- Primary achalasia is a primary motility disorder with 90% of patients reporting dysphagia.
- The esophagus is dilated and fills with contrast.
- The "bird's beak" appearance is a classic finding.
- Corkscrew appearance with spastic contractions and aperistalsis is supportive.
- Filling defects or mucosal masses, and asymmetry in the contrast column in the strictured area suggest malignancy.
- Secondary achalasia has a shorter duration of symptoms. Chagas disease is an infection caused by the protozoan *Trypanosoma cruzi* that results in achalasia
- Treatment is with pneumatic dilation, botulinum toxin, or myotomy.

■ **Other Imaging Findings**

- Whereas cross-sectional imaging can detect esophageal dilation, evaluation of the stricture is best done by a barium esophagram.

✓ **Pearls and** ✗ **Pitfalls**

- ✓ Multiple views should be obtained to ensure there is no underlying mass.
- ✓ A tram-track appearance of the strictured segment suggests primary achalasia.
- ✗ Debris in the obstructed esophagus can obscure lesions.
- ✗ Long-segment strictures are more likely to be due to secondary achalasia.

Case 74

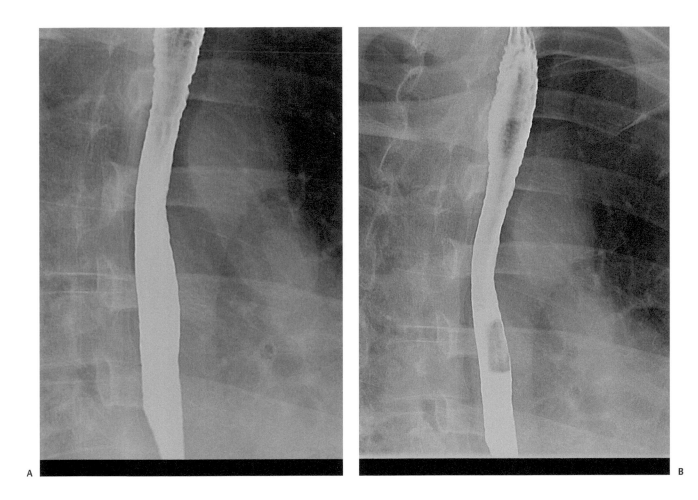

A   B

■ Clinical Presentation

A 32-year-old male with dysphagia when swallowing solid foods.

■ **Imaging Findings**

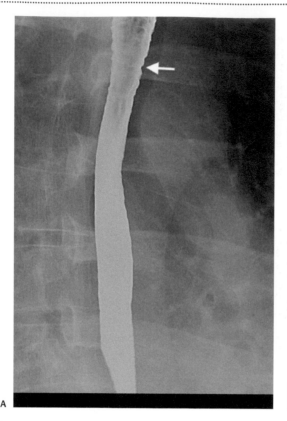
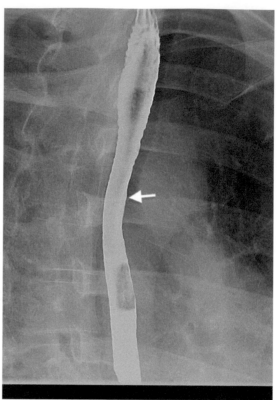

(A) Double-contrast barium esophagram shows fine rings in the proximal esophagus (*arrow*). **(B)** Double-contrast barium esophagram shows a narrowed esophagus that persists with proximal rings (*arrow*).

■ **Differential Diagnosis**

- ***Eosinophilic esophagitis:*** Inflammatory disorder of the esophagus associated with atopy.
- *Chronic reflux esophagitis:* Inflammation caused by gastrointestinal reflux.

■ **Essential Facts**

- Eosinophilic esophagitis is inflammation of the esophagus with eosinophilic infiltration of the esophageal mucosa.
- Esophagram will show multiple concentric rings in the proximal esophagus.
- Segmental strictures and midesophageal narrowing can be present.
- The esophagus is diffusely small in caliber.
- Radiography is more accurate than endoscopy to identify strictures.
- Normal esophagus should have a maximal diameter of 20 mm and a minimal diameter of 15 mm.

■ **Other Imaging Findings**

- Single-contrast exam can be used in certain cases to document strictures but may not show the mucosal findings.

✓ **Pearls and** ✗ **Pitfalls**

- ✓ Evaluate for persistent strictures or narrowing.
- ✓ Proximal ringed esophagus is persistent through the esophagram.
- ✗ Nonpersistent transverse (feline esophagus) folds are associated with reflux disease.
- ✗ Long-segment strictures with longitudinal folds or web-like strictures can indicate Barrett's esophagus.

Case 75

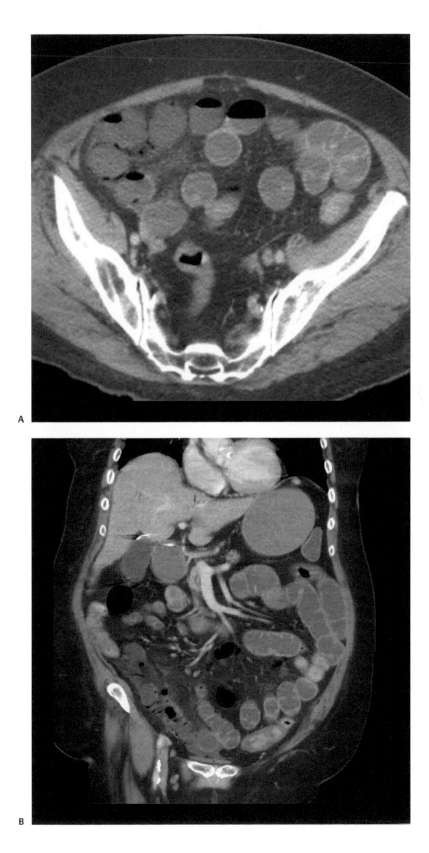

■ Clinical Presentation

A 60-year-old patient with severe abdominal pain.

■ Imaging Findings

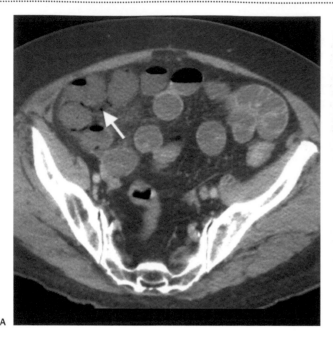 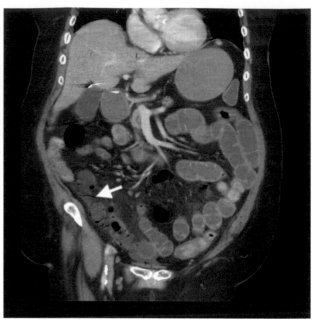

A   B

(A) Axial contrast-enhanced computed tomography (CT) shows dilated loops of small bowel and bowel wall pneumatosis (*arrow*); poor wall enhancement is noted in the right lower quadrant. **(B)** Coronal contrast-enhanced CT shows dilated loops of small bowel with bowel wall pneumatosis and free air (*arrow*).

■ Differential Diagnosis

• ***Bowel obstruction with ischemia of the ilium.***

■ Essential Facts

• Most common cause of bowel obstruction is adhesive disease, followed by hernias and malignancies.
• Two-view plain film radiographs have a reported sensitivity, specificity, and accuracy of 82%, 83%, and 83%, respectively.
• Specific CT findings are small bowel dilated ≥ 2.5 cm and colon not dilated.
• Transition point from dilated to nondilated small bowel is supportive.
• Ischemic changes in the bowel include bowel wall thickening, pneumatosis, poor enhancement, mesenteric edema, attenuated or occluded vessels, and free air.

■ Other Imaging Findings

• Two-view abdominal radiographs can be used as a test when evaluating for small bowel obstruction (SBO).
• Magnetic resonance imaging has a limited role in the setting of acute SBO.

✓ Pearls and ✗ Pitfalls

✓ Intravenous contrast helps evaluate bowel wall enhancement and vessel opacification for ischemia.
✓ The small bowel feces sign occurs immediately proximal to the level of obstruction and helps detect the site of obstruction.
✗ Partial SBO can be difficult to accurately detect.
✗ Early signs of ischemia can be subtle with mild perfusion changes and mesenteric edema.

Case 76

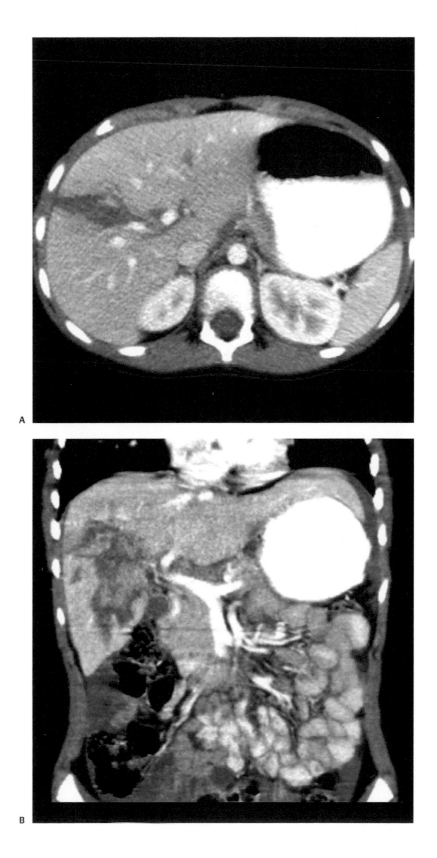

A

B

■ Clinical Presentation

A teenager with abdominal pain after a bicycle accident: follow-up computed tomography (CT) exam.

■ Imaging Findings

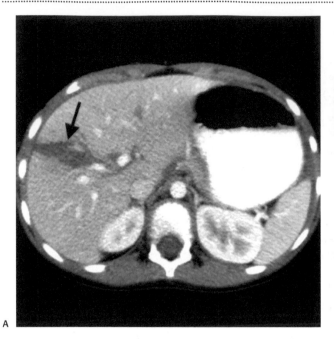 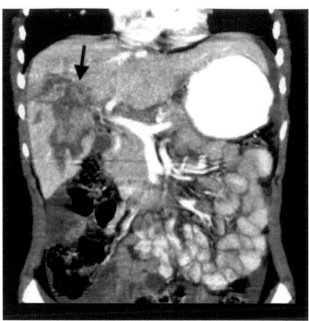

(A) Axial contrast-enhanced computed tomography (CT) shows a laceration extending from the capsule to the hilum about the hepatic vessels (*arrow*). The laceration is > 3 cm in depth and > 10 cm in length (grade III). (B) Coronal contrast-enhanced CT shows the branching laceration extending down the right hepatic lobe (*arrow*). No active contrast extravasation is present.

■ Differential Diagnosis

- **Hepatic laceration:** Liver injury caused by blunt force or penetrating trauma. It may involve the hepatic vessels and biliary tree and be associated with active bleeding.

■ Essential Facts

- Hepatic lacerations may occur from either penetrating or blunt force trauma.
- American Association for the Surgery of Trauma organ injury grading is from I to V based on vascular injury and laceration.
- Grade I: subcapsular hematoma < 10% surface area; parenchymal laceration < 1 cm depth; capsular tear.
- Grade II: subcapsular hematoma 10–50% surface area; intraparenchymal hematoma; < 10 cm in diameter; laceration 1–3 cm in depth and ≤ 10 cm length.
- Grade III: subcapsular hematoma > 50% surface area; ruptured subcapsular or parenchymal hematoma; intraparenchymal hematoma >10 cm; laceration > 3 cm depth; any injury in the presence of a liver vascular injury or active bleeding contained within liver parenchyma.
- Grade IV: parenchymal disruption involving 25–75% of a hepatic lobe; active bleeding extending beyond the liver parenchyma into the peritoneum.
- Grade V: parenchymal disruption > 75% of hepatic lobe; juxtahepatic venous injury to include retrohepatic vena cava and central major hepatic veins.

■ Other Imaging Findings

- CT is the imaging choice for trauma.
- Ultrasound has limited role in detection of perihepatic fluid, pseudoaneurysm, and vessel injury.

✓ Pearls and ✗ Pitfalls

✓ Posttraumatic pseudoaneurysm can result in hemobilia.
✓ Proper contrast bolus and timing is necessary to assess active extravasation and hematoma.
✗ Biliary injury may not be evident on the initial CT and may require follow-up exams.
✗ Higher liver injury scores do not necessarily correlate with the need for surgical intervention.

Case 77

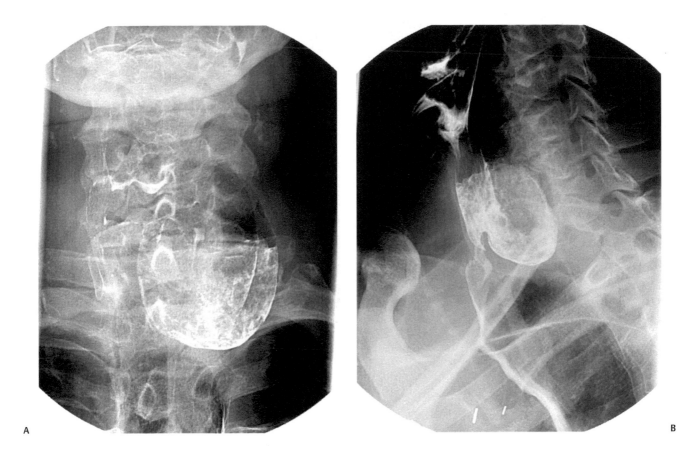

A

B

■ Clinical Presentation

An elderly male with a globus sensation, dysphagia, and halitosis.

■ Imaging Findings

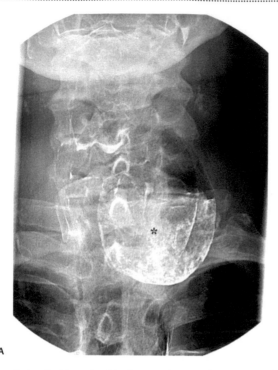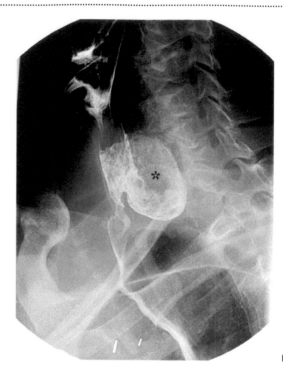

A   **B**

(A) Anteroposterior double-contrast barium esophagram shows a smooth, large outpouching at the level of the hypopharynx that contains semisolid bezoar (*asterisk*). **(B)** Oblique double-contrast barium esophagram shows the diverticulum compressing the esophagus (*asterisk*).

■ Differential Diagnosis

- **Zenker's diverticulum:** Posterior inferior esophageal pseudodiverticulum above the cricopharyngeal muscle.
- *Killian–Jamieson diverticulum:* Typically, small, anterolateral esophageal diverticulum at the level of C5-C6.

■ Essential Facts

- Zenker's diverticulum is the most common diverticulum of the upper gastrointestinal tract.
- Zenker's is a pulsion-pseudodiverticulum resulting in herniation of the pharyngeal mucosa and submucosa between the inferior pharyngeal constrictor (thyropharyngeus) and the horizontal fibers of the cricopharyngeus.
- Zenker's diverticulum is usually located at the midline or left of midline on frontal images and extends posteriorly and inferiorly on lateral images.
- Zenker's can compress the esophagus posteriorly.

■ Other Imaging Findings

- Barium esophagram with cine fluoroscopy is the screening test of choice as it is dynamic, is easy to perform, and has good accuracy.

✓ Pearls and ✗ Pitfalls

- ✓ Obtain cine images in both the frontal and lateral projections.
- ✓ Zenker's is associated with esophageal webs.
- ✗ A prominent cricopharyngeus muscle may mimic the appearance of a diverticulum.
- ✗ Small diverticula or transient outpouchings that fill and empty can be missed if cine fluoroscopy is not used.

Case 78

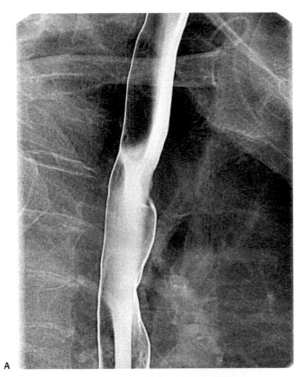

A

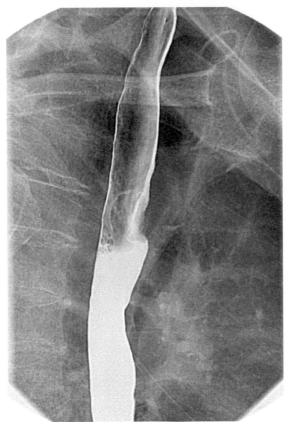

B

■ Clinical Presentation

A 70-year-old female with dysphagia.

■ **Imaging Findings**

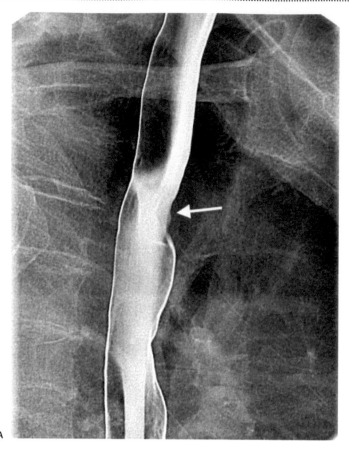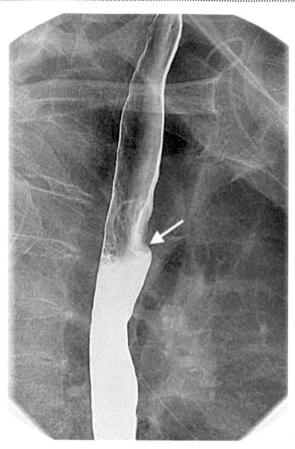

A   B

(A) Double-contrast barium esophagram shows a upper-esophageal mucosal lesion with an ulceration (*arrow*). Note the focal asymmetric stricture. The proximal margin is tapered. **(B)** Double-contrast barium esophagram shows the outline of the irregularly contoured mucosal mass (*arrow*). The distal margin is shelf-like.

■ **Differential Diagnosis**

- **Esophageal carcinoma:** Carcinoma arising from the mucosa of the esophagus.
- *Esophageal stricture:* Ulceration of the mucosa of the esophagus resulting in a stricture.

■ **Essential Facts**

- Barium esophagram is an inexpensive, relatively accurate method of evaluating suspected esophageal obstruction.
- Features of malignant stricturing include asymmetric narrowing, shelf-like margins, irregular contour, and a nodular or ulcerated mucosal surface.
- Features of a benign stricture include symmetric narrowing, tapered margins, a smooth contour, and a smooth mucosal surface.
- Computed tomography (CT) or positron emission tomography/CT is needed to stage the disease as nodal spread occurs early.

■ **Other Imaging Findings**

- CT is a poor modality for detecting small mucosal lesions.

✓ **Pearls and ✗ Pitfalls**

- ✓ Obtain double-contrast images in two orthogonal planes.
- ✓ Use of a barium tablet can help determine the size of the lumen.
- ✗ Single-contrast esophagram or poor distention can miss mucosal lesions.
- ✗ Gastroesophageal lesions require additional views such as a right lateral decubitus view.

Case 79

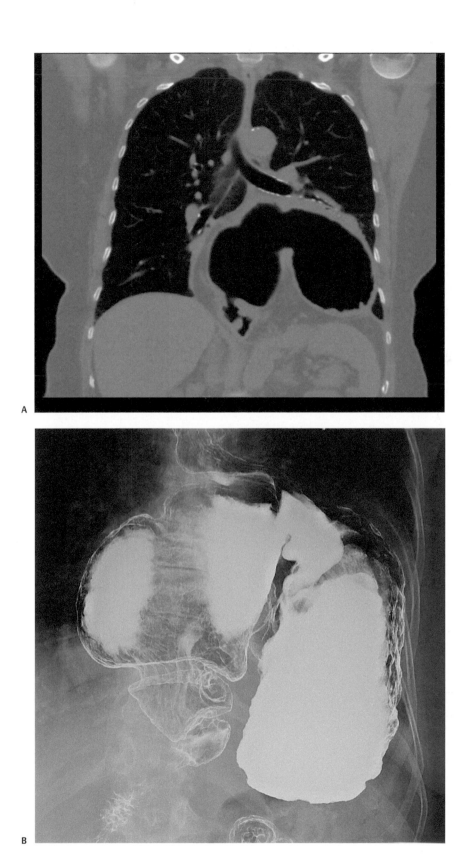

A

B

■ Clinical Presentation

An elderly female presents with chest and abdominal pain.

■ Imaging Findings

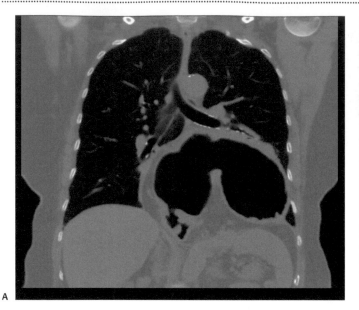
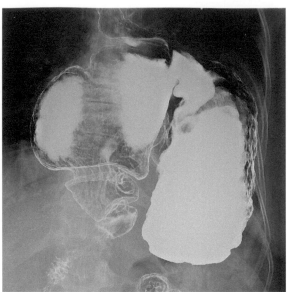

A   B

(A) Coronal computed tomography (CT) shows a diaphragmatic eventration with an intrathoracic stomach. The antrum and pylorus have rotated superiorly and the fundus inferiorly. **(B)** Double-contrast upper gastrointestinal exam shows the intrathoracic stomach with organoaxial volvulus.

■ Differential Diagnosis

- ***Organoaxial gastric volvulus:*** Volvulus along the long axis of the stomach.
- *Mesenteroaxial gastric volvulus:* Volvulus across the short axis of the stomach.
- *Combined type:* A combination of organo- and mesenteroaxial volvulus.

■ Essential Facts

- In organoaxial gastric volvulus, the antrum and pylorus rotate anterosuperiorly and the fundus rotates posterioinferiorly.
- Peak age is in the fifth decade of life.
- Organoaxial gastric volvulus represents ~60% of gastric volvulus and is associated with para-esophageal hernias and diaphragmatic eventration.
- Necrosis and perforation are complications in cases where rotation exceeds 180 degrees.

■ Other Imaging Findings

- Barium upper gastrointestinal imaging is an accurate method of detecting gastric volvulus (80%).
- CT is also good for evaluating volvulus, particularly gastric anatomy and associated complications.

✓ Pearls and ✗ Pitfalls

- ✓ Organoaxial gastric volvulus is frequently associated with diaphragmatic hernia or eventration.
- ✓ Coronal CT and the position of the nasogastric tube can help in evaluation.
- ✗ Changes in gastric position in the setting of chronic gastric volvulus can result in obstruction.
- ✗ Early gastric ischemia can be difficult to detect.

Case 80

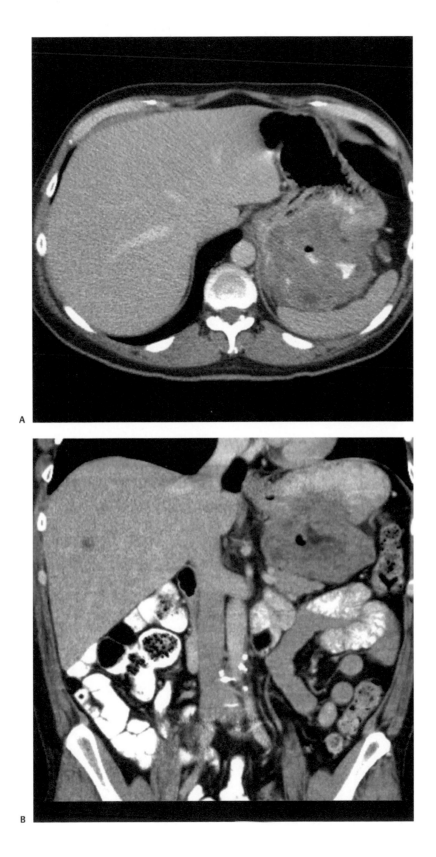

A

B

■ Clinical Presentation

A 72-year-old male presents with weight loss and anemia.

■ Imaging Findings

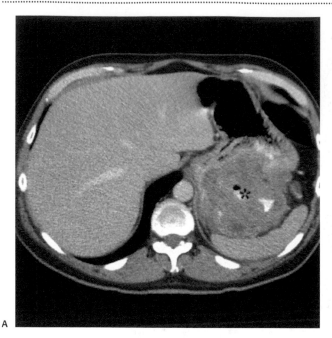
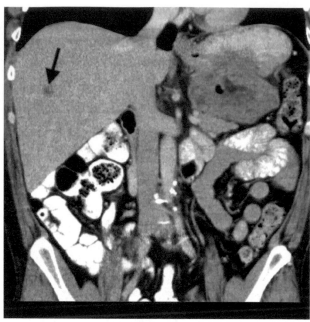

(A) Axial computed tomography (CT) shows a large, partially necrotic mass in the stomach with central necrosis that fills with oral contrast (*asterisk*). **(B)** Coronal CT shows a gastric mass and a focal lesion in the liver (*arrow*). Note the position of the mass with an endoluminal and exophytic component.

■ Differential Diagnosis

- **Gastric gastrointestinal stromal tumor (GIST):** Rare mesenchymal tumor of the stomach.
- *Gastric adenocarcinoma:* Mucosal carcinoma of the stomach.

■ Essential Facts

- GISTs account for 90% of mesenchymal tumors in the gastrointestinal tract and 2–3% of all gastric malignancies.
- Areas of hemorrhage, necrosis, or cystic degeneration are common, appearing as focal areas of low attenuation.
- Gastric GISTs < 2 cm in size may have no or extremely low malignant potential.
- GIST origin in the stomach is a favorable prognostic factor.
- Focal ulceration is common due to pressure necrosis.
- Metastasis is most commonly to the liver and peritoneum.

■ Other Imaging Findings

- Magnetic resonance enterography or barium upper gastrointestinal imaging can be used to evaluate the stomach for masses. Purely exophytic masses without any ulceration can be missed on barium upper gastrointestinal imaging.

✓ Pearls and ✗ Pitfalls

- ✓ Large rounded necrotic masses in the stomach are characteristic of GISTs.
- ✓ Look for liver and peritoneal metastases as they are common.
- ✗ Gastric GISTs can be difficult to detect in a collapsed stomach.
- ✗ Variety of other gastric mesenchymal masses such as leiomyomas, schwannomas, hemangiomas, inflammatory myofibroblastic tumors, and carcinoids can mimic GIST and cannot be differentiated by imaging.

Case 81

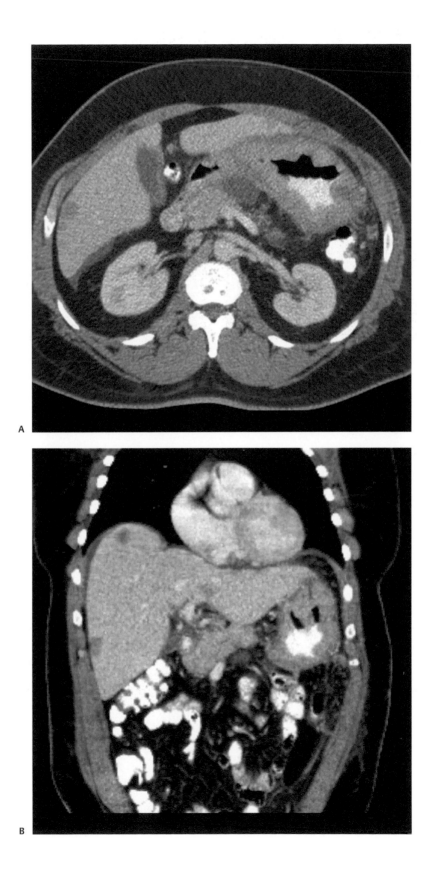

A

B

■ Clinical Presentation

A 65-year-old male presents with weight loss and anemia.

■ Imaging Findings

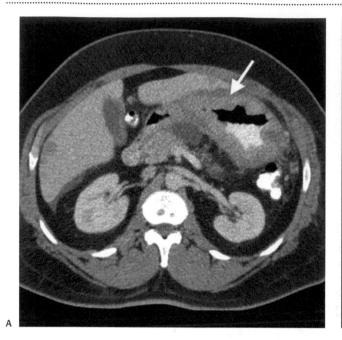 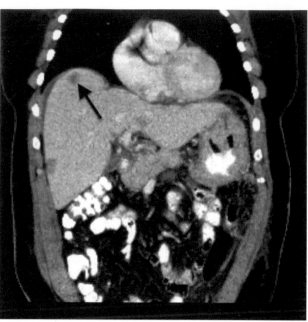

A   B

(A) Axial contrast-enhanced computed tomography (CT) shows diffuse gastric-wall thickening with peritoneal nodularity in the left upper abdomen and liver lesions (*arrow*). **(B)** Coronal contrast-enhanced CT shows fundal wall thickening and liver lesions (*arrow*).

■ Differential Diagnosis

- *Gastric carcinoma:* Carcinoma of the stomach mucosa; most gastric cancers are adenocarcinomas of mucous cell origin.
- *Gastric lymphoma:* Primary lymphoma of the stomach either mucosa-associated lymphoid tissue gastric lymphoma or diffuse large B-cell lymphoma.

■ Essential Facts

- Imaging features of gastric carcinoma depending on the morphologic type: polypoid, fungating, ulcerated, infiltrative (Borrmann types I to IV).
- In transmural disease, the serosal contour is blurred.
- Gastric carcinoma spreads to the liver via the gastrohepatic ligament, the colon via the gastrocolic ligament, and the pancreas via the lesser sac.
- Distal esophagus is directly involved in tumors of the cardia in 60%.

- Duodenum is involved in ~15% of patients with antral disease.
- Lymphatic spread is common in gastric carcinoma.

■ Other Imaging Findings

- Positron emission tomography/CT is an excellent modality to detect and stage gastric carcinoma as most lesions are fluorodeoxyglucose avid.

✓ Pearls and ✗ Pitfalls

- ✓ Mucosal lesions can be detected with appropriate gastric distention.
- ✓ Infiltration of the perigastric fat or blurring of the serosal contour indicates transmural disease.
- ✗ Gastric ulcers and gastritis can mimic gastric carcinoma.
- ✗ Evaluation of the distal antrum and gastric cardia is difficult as these segments are frequently not distended.

Case 82

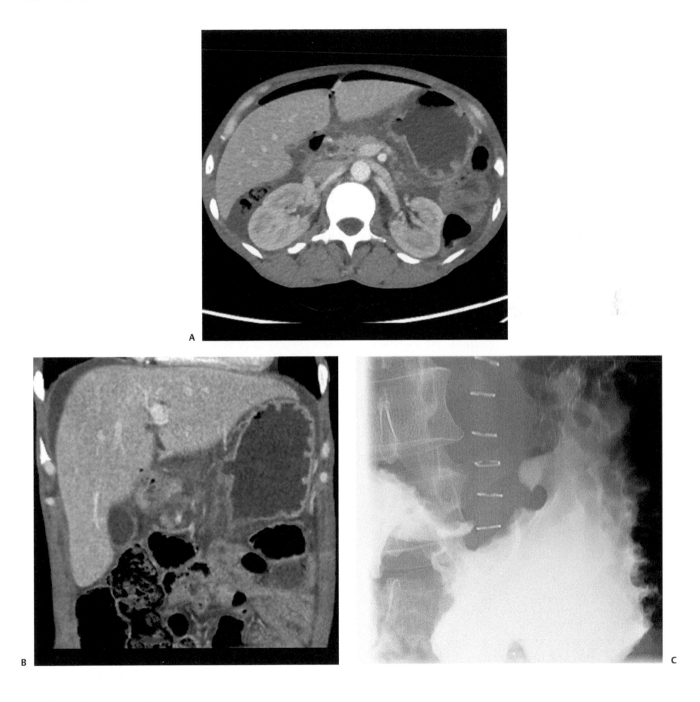

■ Clinical Presentation

A 45-year-old intravenous drug user presents with excruciating abdominal pain.

■ **Imaging Findings**

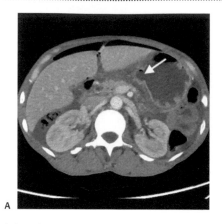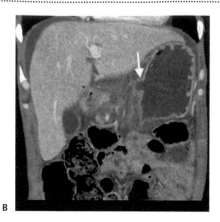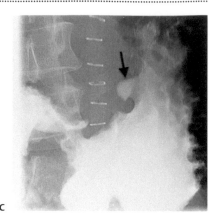

A   B   C

(A) Axial contrast-enhanced computed tomography (CT) shows extensive upper abdominal free air and free fluid (*arrow*). Focal mucosal ulcer is noted along the lesser curvature of the stomach. **(B)** Coronal contrast-enhanced CT shows a well-demarcated ulceration in the lesser curvature with submucosal edema (*arrow*); the base is smooth and has a regular edge. **(C)** Upper gastrointestinal imaging shows a focal ulcer in the lesser curvature of the stomach that is deep to the mucosal surface of the stomach (*arrow*).

■ **Differential Diagnosis**

- ***Benign gastric ulcer:*** Mucosal ulceration secondary to gastric acid.
- *Malignant gastric ulcer:* Ulcerated gastric cancer, most commonly ulcerated adenocarcinoma.

■ **Essential Facts**

- Risk factors for peptic ulcer disease are *Helicobacter pylori*, nonsteroidal anti-inflammatory drug use, smoking, and physiologic stress.
- On CT, there is preservation of the submucosal fat layer in benign gastric ulcers.
- Benign gastric ulcers have smooth and regular shapes, even bases, clearly demarcated and regular edges, and folds that taper and converge toward the ulcer.

■ **Other Imaging Findings**

- On upper gastrointestinal imaging, benign gastric ulcers project beyond the gastric mucosa, have a smooth ulcer collar, and have thick gastric folds that can radiate to the base of the ulcer.

✓ **Pearls and** ✗ **Pitfalls**

- ✓ Preservation of the submucosal fat is a sign the ulcer is benign.
- ✓ A smooth ulcer deep to the gastric mucosa without a mass is a sign the ulcer is benign.
- ✗ About 6% of gastric ulcers are malignant and need endoscopic follow-up.
- ✗ Contracted stomach with hypoattenuating mural thickening may mimic peptic ulcer disease.

Case 83

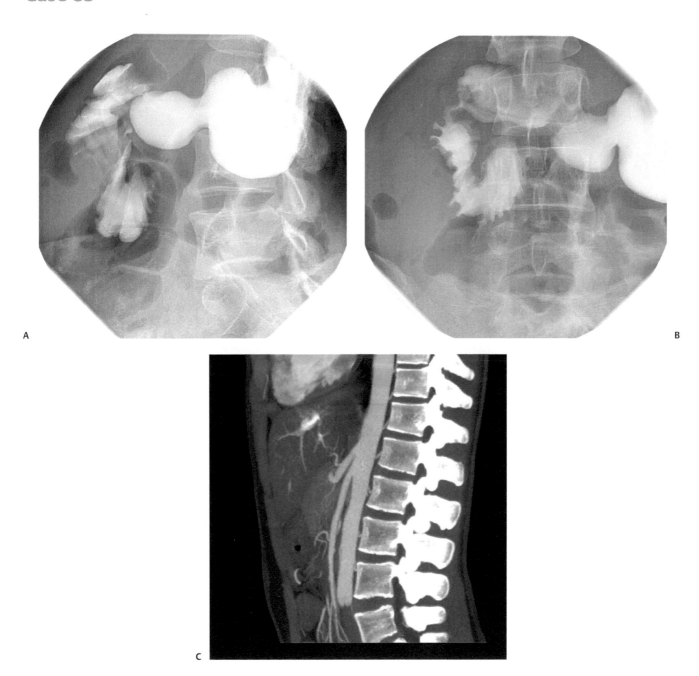

A

B

C

■ Clinical Presentation

A 39-year-old female with postprandial pain and weight loss.

■ **Imaging Findings**

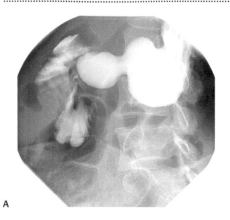 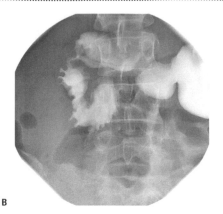 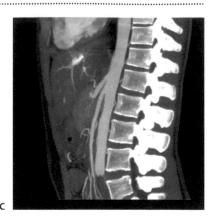

A   B   C

(A) Barium study shows well-distended duodenum to midline. **(B)** Barium study shows cutoff of the contrast column at midline. Cine fluoroscopy showed antiperistaltic flow of the contrast column proximal to the site of obstruction. **(C)** Sagittal computed tomography (CT) angiography shows narrow aorto-mesenteric angle and low aortomesenteric distance causing compression of the duodenum by the superior mesenteric artery (SMA).

■ **Differential Diagnosis**

- ***Superior mesenteric artery compression syndrome:*** Compression of the transverse portion of the duodenum by the superior mesenteric artery.
- *Obstructive duodenal mass:* Duodenal mass, either benign or malignant, that obstructs the duodenum.

■ **Essential Facts**

- Compression of the transverse portion of the duodenum by the superior mesenteric artery is also known as Wilkie's syndrome or Cast syndrome.
- Patients have an acute aortomesenteric angle < 22 degrees; normal angle is 25 to 60 degrees.
- The aortomesenteric distance is reduced to 8 to 10 mm; normal is 10 to 28 mm.
- The duodenum is suspended by the ligament of Treitz; a high fixation is considered a predisposing factor.
- Can be a sequelae of weight loss with loss of the mesenteric fat pad.
- Can be the result of corrective scoliosis procedure that lengthens the spine and narrows the aortomesenteric angle resulting in SMA compression.

■ **Other Imaging Findings**

- Sagittal plane CT is used to measure the aortomesenteric angle and distance.

✓ **Pearls and** ✗ **Pitfalls**

- ✓ Cine fluoroscopy should be used to image the first passage of contrast in the duodenum.
- ✓ Placing the patient prone or in the left lateral position relieves the symptoms.
- ✗ An acute aortomesenteric angle may not always produce signs of compression.
- ✗ SMA compression syndrome is a diagnosis of exclusion. Other entities can produce similar symptoms.

Case 84

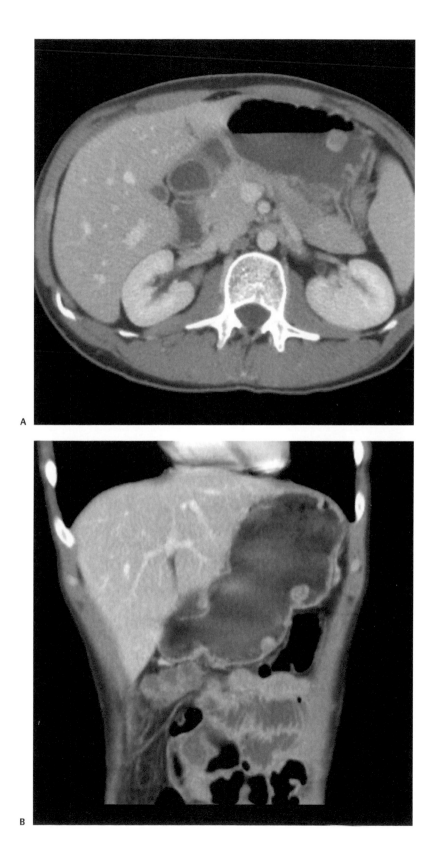

A

B

■ Clinical Presentation

A young male with anemia undergoes computed tomography (CT) enterography.

■ Imaging Findings

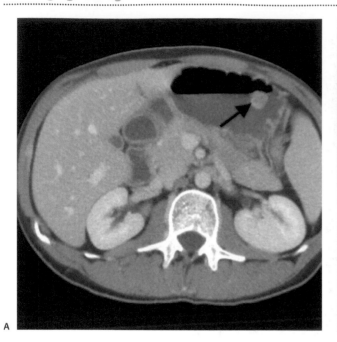
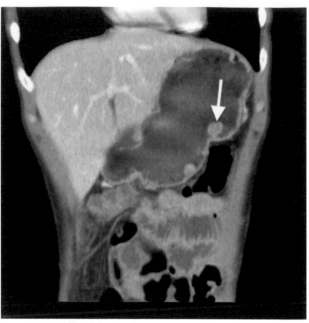

(A) Axial contrast-enhanced CT shows a polyp in the gastric body (*arrow*). **(B)** Coronal contrast-enhanced CT shows multiple polyps in the stomach with normal-appearing adjacent mucosa (*arrow*).

■ Differential Diagnosis

- ***Peutz–Jeghers polyps:*** Autosomal dominant condition characterized by hamartomatous polyps (Peutz–Jeghers type).
- *Familial adenomatous polyposis:* Autosomal dominant condition with gastric fundic gland polyps with or without dysplasia.
- *Juvenile polyposis:* Autosomal dominant condition with hamartomatous polyps.
- *Cronkhite–Canada syndrome:* Sporadic-inheritance condition characterized by hamartomatous polyps (juvenile type).
- *Cowden/PTEN hamartoma tumor syndrome:* Autosomal dominant characterized by hamartomatous polyps.

■ Essential Facts

- Peutz–Jeghers syndrome (PJS) is an autosomal dominant disease.
- Patients with PJS have small bowel polyps (64%), colonic polyps (53%), and gastric polyps (15–30%).
- A high risk of various malignancies necessitates periodic screening.
- PJS is associated with acute gastrointestinal bleeding, intussusception, and bowel obstruction.

■ Other Imaging Findings

- Magnetic resonance enterography and CT enteroclysis are used for screening of patients.

✓ Pearls and ✗ Pitfalls

- ✓ CT enterography with a neutral contrast agent and good bowel distention is needed to identify polyps.
- ✓ Scrutinize the exam for other PJS-associated gastrointestinal malignancies such as gastric, small bowel, pancreatic, colorectal, and esophageal.
- ✗ Imaging alone cannot exclude malignancy in a particular polyp.
- ✗ Viewing the images in one plane alone can miss polyps that are associated with small bowel folds.

Case 85

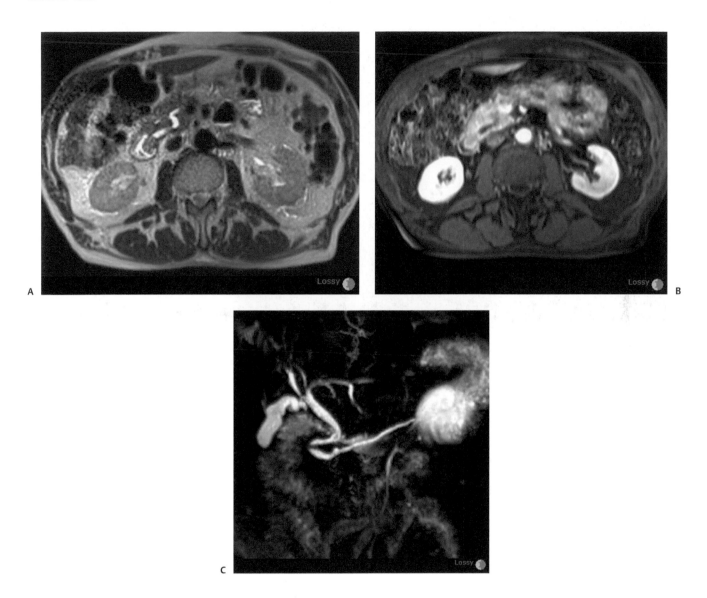

▪ Clinical Presentation

An 80-year-old patient with jaundice and weight loss.

■ **Imaging Findings**

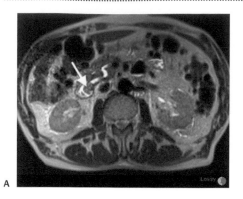 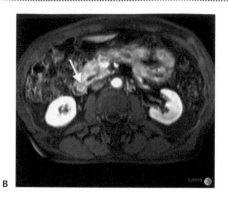 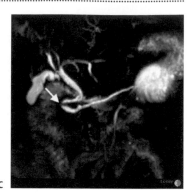

A B C

(A) Axial T2 shows a soft tissue mass at the level of the ampulla (*arrow*). **(B)** Axial T1+C fast spoiled gradient echo shows a small enhancing mass at the ampulla in the duodenum (*arrow*). **(C)** Coronal T2 magnetic resonance cholangiopancreatography (MRCP) shows obstruction of both the common bile duct (CBD) and the main pancreatic duct at the level of the duodenum (*arrow*). Note the smooth tapering of both ducts without an intraductal mass.

■ **Differential Diagnosis**

- ***Ampullary carcinoma:*** Carcinoma affecting the ampulla of Vater located in the major duodenal papilla surrounded by the sphincter of Oddi.
- *Pancreatic carcinoma:* Carcinoma arising from the pancreas, most commonly an adenocarcinoma.

■ **Essential Facts**

- Most ampullary carcinomas are adenocarcinomas arising from the ampulla.
- Ampullary carcinomas produce bulging of the papilla with a mass (62%).
- The distal CBD wall is smooth.
- There is distention and abrupt narrowing of the CBD.
- The intrahepatic ducts are dilated.
- The pancreatic duct may be dilated.
- Prognosis is better than periampullary masses.

■ **Other Imaging Findings**

- Magnetic resonance imaging shows a discrete nodular mass at the distal margin of the pancreaticobiliary junction that is hypointense on T2-weighted imaging and enhances following gadolinium-based contrast agent administration. Diffusion-weighted imaging is useful in identifying the mass.
- On MRCP, the ductal dilation and abrupt tapering are evident.

✓ **Pearls and ✗ Pitfalls**

✓ Distention of the duodenum helps detect ampullary and periampullary masses.

✓ Abrupt narrowing of the CBD is a sign of an ampullary carcinoma.

✗ Ampullary carcinoma and benign ampullary stenosis can cause duodenal wall thickening.

✗ Periampullary masses such as distal CBD cholangiocarcinoma can mimic an ampullary carcinoma.

Case 86

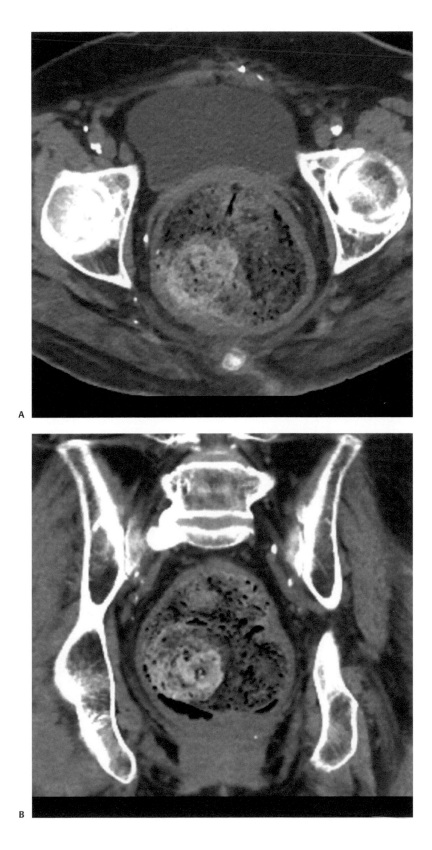

■ Clinical Presentation

A 75-year-old female presents with constipation and abdominal pain.

▪ Imaging Findings

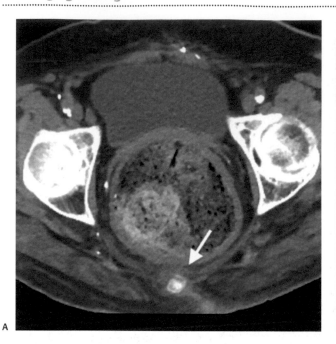
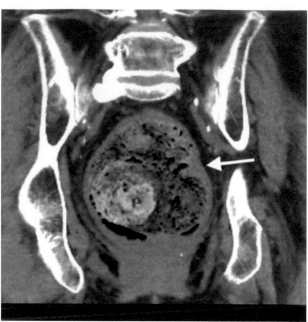

(A) Axial contrast-enhanced computed tomography (CT) shows wall thickening of a distended rectum with scybala (hardened lumps of feces) and presacral edema (*arrow*). (B) Coronal contrast-enhanced CT shows wall thickening of the rectum, which is filled with stool (*arrow*). Note the edema along the inferior aspect.

▪ Differential Diagnosis

- **Fecal impaction and stercoral colitis (SC):** SC is an inflammatory process involving the colonic wall related to fecal impaction.
- *Anorectal cancer:* Anorectal cancers are typically adenocarcinomas, whereas anal cancers are squamous in origin.

▪ Essential Facts

- Fecal impaction can lead to SC.
- There is distention of the colonic lumen, colonic wall thickening, ulceration, and ultimately perforation.
- Common sites of perforation are the peritoneal reflection, the antimesenteric border of the rectosigmoid junction, and the apex of the sigmoid colon.
- In SC, the colon is distended > 6 cm.
- In SC, the rectal wall is thickened > 3 mm.
- Discontinuous mucosa or free air are findings of perforation.
- Hyperdense mucosa indicates hemorrhage.

▪ Other Imaging Findings

- Plain film radiographs of the abdomen would show feces in a distended rectum. There may be proximal colonic distention.

✓ Pearls and ✗ Pitfalls

- ✓ Colonic wall thickening and surrounding fat infiltration are indicators of colitis.
- ✓ Hyperdense mucosa results from mucosal hemorrhage and indicates the process is severe.
- ✗ Patients with Ogilvie's syndrome can have significant colonic distention > 10 cm.
- ✗ Colonic perforation may be sealed off by a fecaloma or inflammatory fibrin and may not produce free air.

Case 87

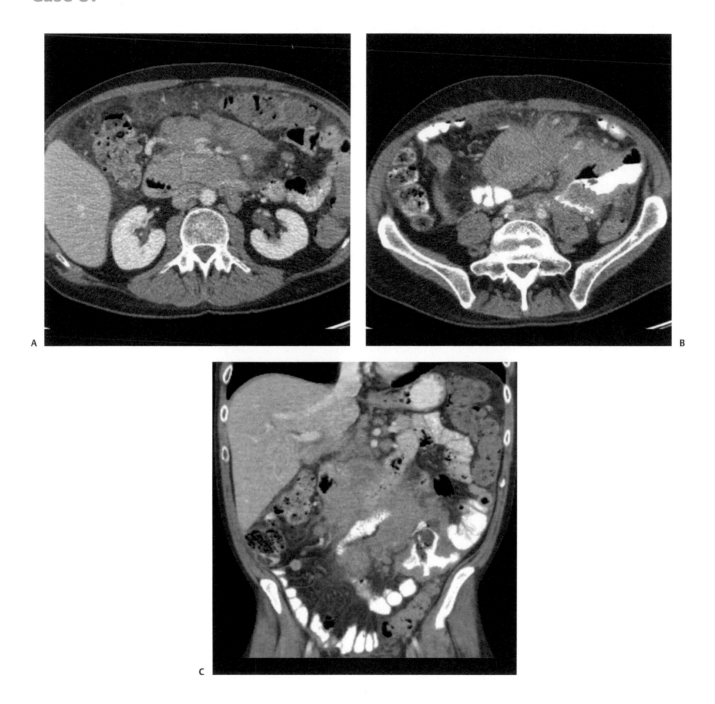

A

B

C

■ **Clinical Presentation**

A 50-year-old male presents with weight loss and night sweats.

■ Imaging Findings

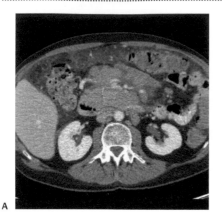 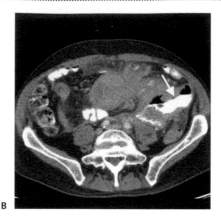 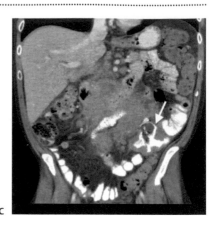

A   B   C

(A) Axial contrast-enhanced computed tomography (CT) shows diffuse mesenteric adenopathy about the mesenteric vessels. **(B)** Axial contrast-enhanced CT shows soft tissue involvement of the small bowel with focal aneurysmal dilation (*arrow*). **(C)** Coronal contrast-enhanced CT shows extensive soft tissue involvement of the mesentery and small bowel with focal bowel dilation and fistula formation (*arrow*).

■ Differential Diagnosis

• **Lymphoma of the small bowel:** Lymphomatous involvement of the small bowel can occur as either primary small bowel lymphoma or secondary involvement (extranodal involvement).
• *Carcinoma of the small bowel:* Adenocarcinoma of the small bowel most commonly affects the duodenum and jejunum, except for cases of Crohn's disease, which most commonly arise in the ileum.

■ Essential Facts

• B-cell lymphoma is the most common type that affects the bowel, and the stomach is the most common site affected.
• T-cell lymphoma is associated with celiac disease and occurs most commonly in the jejunum.
• Epstein-Barr virus (EBV) has an association with Burkitt's lymphoma, which commonly occurs in the ileocecal region in pediatric patients.
• The most common lymphoma patterns are polypoid/ nodular, infiltrative, aneurysmal, exophytic mass, and, rarely, stenosing mass.
• Small, polypoid masses can be a lead point for intussusception.
• Small bowel lymphoma rarely presents with obstruction.
• Risk factors include immunodeficiency syndrome, inflammatory bowel disease, immunosuppression after solid organ transplantation, systemic lupus erythematosus, and chemotherapy.

■ Other Imaging Findings

• Magnetic resonance (MR) enterography is good for evaluating lymphoma involving the bowel. Lymphoma usually has homogeneous intermediate signal intensity on T1-weighted MR images and heterogeneous high signal intensity on T2-weighted imaging. Mild to moderate enhancement is seen after the intravenous administration of gadolinium-based contrast material.

✓ Pearls and ✗ Pitfalls

✓ Nodal disease is more bulky in cases of lymphoma compared with adenocarcinoma.
✓ Disease spread into the fat that manifests as fat infiltration is more common with small bowel adenocarcinoma.
✗ Small polypoid masses in the bowel or stomach may not be detected without adequate bowel distention.
✗ Lymphoma of the terminal ileum can mimic Crohn's disease.

Case 88

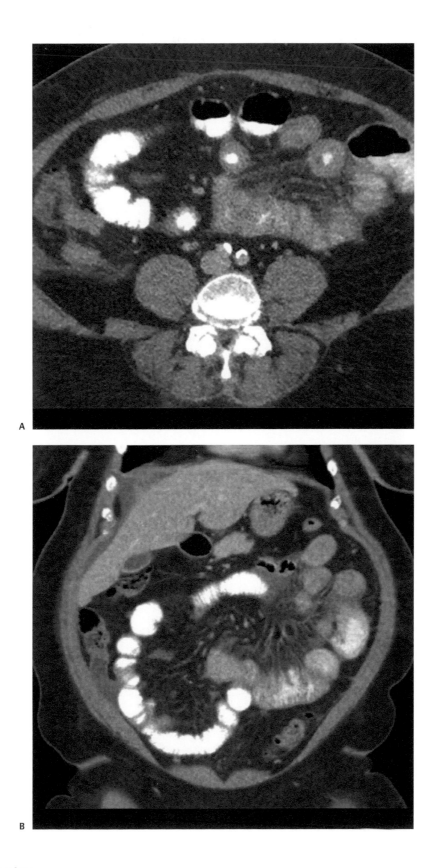

A

B

■ **Clinical Presentation**

A 65-year-old female with hypertension presents with abdominal pain and diarrhea.

■ Imaging Findings

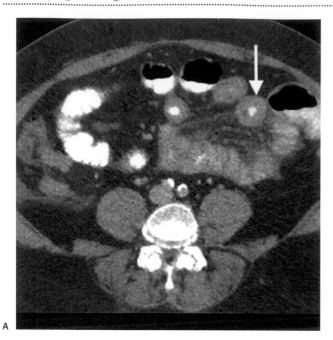 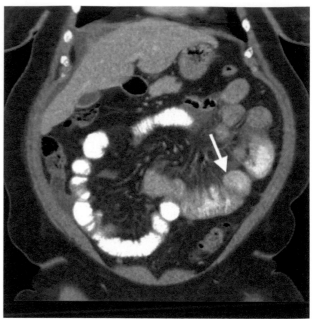

(A) Axial contrast-enhanced computed tomography (CT) shows diffuse bowel wall thickening with submucosal edema of the jejunum with engorged vessels (*arrow*). **(B)** Coronal contrast-enhanced CT shows diffuse jejunal wall thickening with mesenteric edema and some ascites (*arrow*). Note the contrast transits the involved bowel segment.

■ Differential Diagnosis

- ***Angiotensin-converting enzyme (ACE) inhibitor-induced angioedema:*** A drug-induced angioedema that affects the face, mouth, upper airway, and small bowel.
- *Small bowel enteritis:* Nonspecific enteritis that can be infectious, inflammatory, or due to ischemia.

■ Essential Facts

- Incidence of ACE inhibitor–induced angioedema is estimated at approximately 0.3%.
- Contributing factors include a history of allergies, age > 65 years, female, and obesity.
- Presentation can be days to years after medications are initially administered.
- Involves the jejunum only in the majority of the cases followed by ileum only and jejunum plus ileum.

■ Other Imaging Findings

- Magnetic resonance enterography can show the thickened bowel wall with enhancing mucosa—"target sign"—without bowel obstruction.

✓ Pearls and ✗ Pitfalls

- ✓ History of ACE inhibitor use is helpful in making the diagnosis.
- ✓ Disease can be confined to the jejunum without bowel obstruction.
- ✗ Acute mesenteric venous ischemia has similar findings.
- ✗ Vasculitis including systemic lupus erythematosus can mimic angioedema.

Case 89

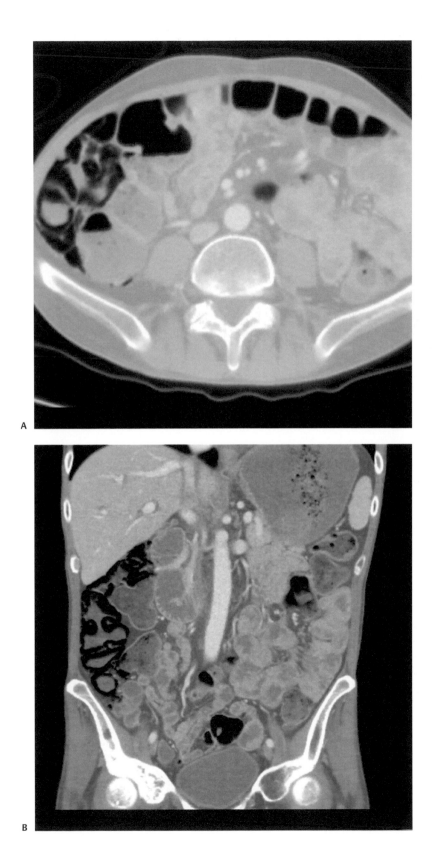

A

B

A 53-year-old male following allogenic stem cell transplant presents with abdominal pain.

■ **Imaging Findings**

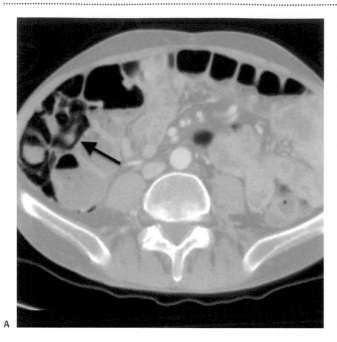 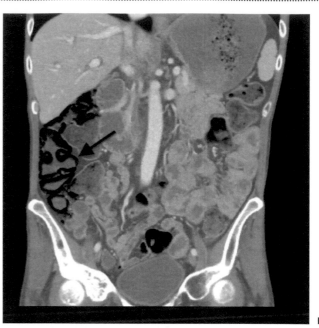

A   B

(A) Axial contrast-enhanced computed tomography (CT) shows pneumatosis intestinalis (PI) with gas in the wall of the ascending colon (*arrow*). **(B)** Coronal contrast-enhanced CT shows gas in wall of the cecum and ascending colon (*arrow*); no bowel obstruction or wall thickening is present.

■ **Differential Diagnosis**

- ***Pneumatosis intestinalis (PI):*** Secondary form with gas in the wall of the small bowel or colon.
- *Pneumatosis cystoides intestinalis:* Primary form with multiple cysts in the colonic submucosa or serosa.

■ **Essential Facts**

- Wall disruption, increased wall permeability, or necrosis leads to wall infiltration by gas.
- Increased intraluminal pressure in the setting of a normal mucosal barrier can lead to PI.
- PI can be seen in the setting of bowel ischemia.
- PI can occur in the setting of celiac disease, connective tissue disorders, systemic lupus erythematosus, infectious enteritis, chronic obstructive pulmonary disease, primary or acquired immunodeficiency syndrome, leukemia, organ transplantation, bone marrow transplantation, and in patients receiving glucocorticoids and chemotherapy.
- PI is associated with a high mortality rate of 33 to 44%.

■ **Other Imaging Findings**

- Sonography is limited for evaluating the bowel. However, it can be used to detect PI in the pediatric patient. PI appears as linear or focal echogenic areas within the bowel wall. It can also appear as a continuous echogenic ring in the bowel wall. Rarely, PI can also be seen on magnetic resonance imaging (MRI). It is seen as collections of air adherent to or within the bowel wall that became more apparent on gradient-echo images due to blooming artifact associated with magnetic field inhomogeneities at air-tissue interfaces.

✓ **Pearls and ✗ Pitfalls**

- ✓ Clinical symptoms and serum lactic acid levels can help to determine that the cause is ischemic.
- ✓ Changes in the wall such as thickening or fat stranding can indicate ischemia.
- ✗ Bowel contents mixed with air or air trapped between mucosal folds can mimic PI.
- ✗ It is difficult to accurately differentiate benign from life-threatening causes of PI based on imaging alone due to overlap in imaging findings.

Case 90

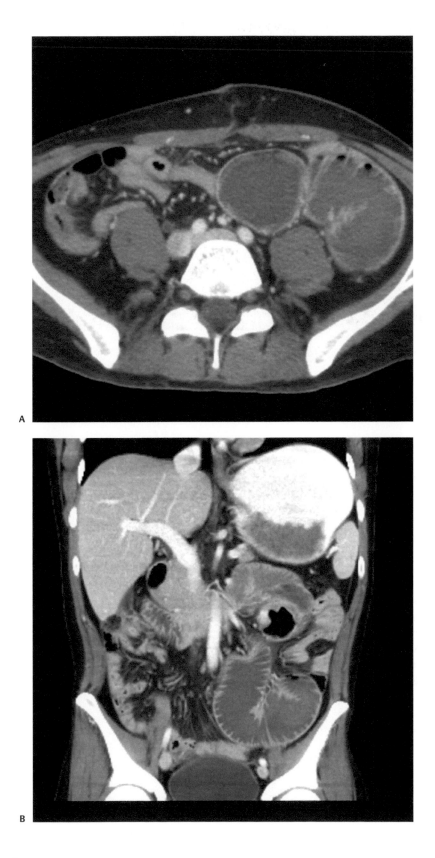

A

B

■ Clinical Presentation

A 44-year-old female with diagnosis of Crohn's enteritis with severe abdominal pain.

■ Imaging Findings

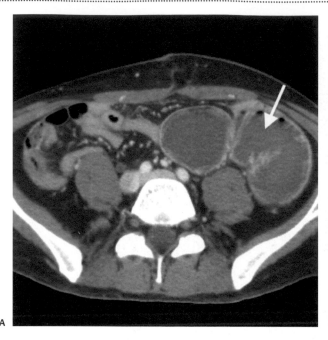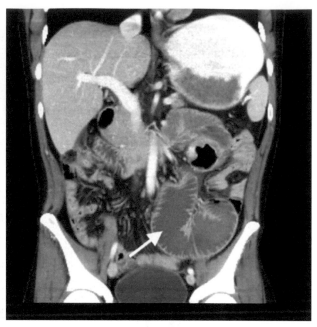

(A) Axial contrast-enhanced computed tomography (CT) shows a cluster of dilated loops in the left lower quadrant and collapsed ileal loops (*arrow*). **(B)** Coronal contrast-enhanced CT shows a fluid-filled loop of bowel in a C-orientation in the left lower abdomen (*arrow*).

■ Differential Diagnosis

- **Closed loop obstruction:** Two points of a section of bowel are obstructed at a single location or adjacent sites, essentially trapping the affected loop.
- *Localized ileus:* Distention of a segment of small bowel without an actual obstruction, commonly caused by adjacent inflammation.

■ Essential Facts

- The most specific CT findings are bowel wall thickening, wall enhancement, and a C- or U-shaped configuration.
- The bowel loops may taper to a point and have interloop fluid.
- When vertically oriented, the obstructed bowel loops can have a radial configuration.
- The afferent and efferent limbs are in close proximity near the site of obstruction.
- Bowel ischemia and perforation is the most severe complication.

■ Other Imaging Findings

- Ultrasound has been used in the evaluation of bowel obstruction. The findings of closed-loop obstruction are an akinetic bowel loop (94%), a hyperechoic and thickened mesentery (82%), and free peritoneal fluid (100%).

✓ Pearls and ✗ Pitfalls

- ✓ Poor wall enhancement, thickened wall, and mesenteric fluid are signs of ischemia.
- ✓ The trapped loop of bowel usually has little to no gas within it.
- ✗ If a large cluster of bowel loops is involved in a closed loop obstruction, the afferent and efferent sites may be hard to identify.
- ✗ Oral contrast may not progress to the site of obstruction as the proximal bowel loops may be fluid filled.

Case 91

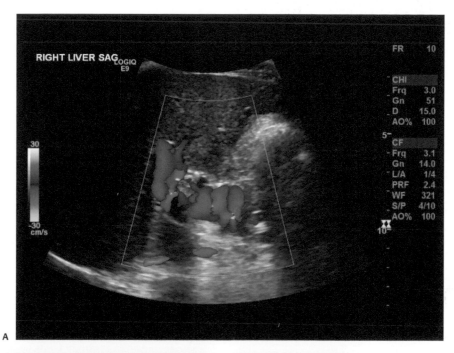

A

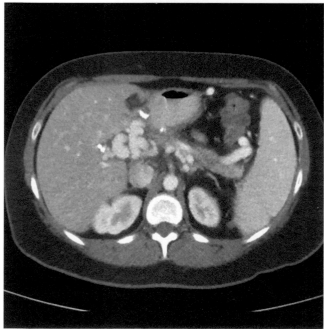

B

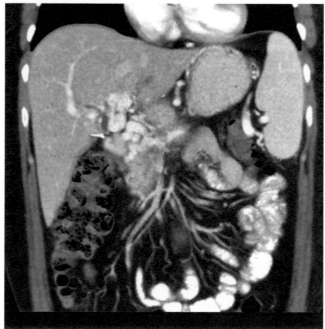

C

■ Clinical Presentation

A 40-year-old female presents with elevated liver enzymes after pancreatitis 3 months ago.

■ Imaging Findings

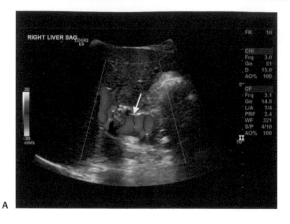
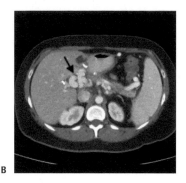
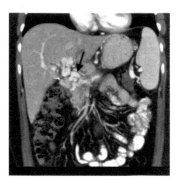

(A) Doppler ultrasound shows multiple vessels at the hepatic hilum in the expected location of the portal vein (*arrow*). **(B)** Axial contrast-enhanced computed tomography (CT) shows a cluster of venous collaterals in the expected location of the main portal vein (*arrow*). **(C)** Coronal contrast-enhanced CT shows the cluster of venous collaterals outside the liver extending from the superior mesenteric vein (*arrow*).

■ Differential Diagnosis

- **Cavernous transformation of the portal vein (CTPV):** Collateral venous drainage formed in the setting of portal vein thrombosis.

■ Essential Facts

- Portal vein thrombosis can be present in the setting of liver disease, abdominal malignancy, infection, and postsurgery.
- CTPV develops 6 to 20 days after the portal venous obstruction occurs.
- CTPV is categorized as either hepatopetal (portal-portal shunts) with venous drainage toward the liver or hepatofugal (portal-systemic shunts) with venous drainage away from the liver.
- Venous collaterals can be periportal or intrahepatic. Portal cavernoma refers to a mass-like or sponge-like appearance of collaterals in some cases.
- Venous collaterals can form in the hepatocolic and hepatoduodenal ligaments, along the gallbladder, and along the peritoneal surface of the liver.
- Complications after development of CTPV include sequelae of portal hypertension, mesenteric congestion and ischemia, portal biliopathy, cholangitis, and biliary cirrhosis.

■ Other Imaging Findings

- Ultrasound is a good screening tool to detect suspected portal venous occlusion and CTPV at the porta hepatis. Various upper abdominal venous collaterals can be detected via ultrasound.
- Magnetic resonance imaging is excellent at detecting portal venous occlusion and collateral formation.

✓ Pearls and ✗ Pitfalls

- ✓ Features of portal hypertension such as splenomegaly and ascites may result from portal vein thrombosis.
- ✓ Magnetic resonance cholangiopancreatography can be performed in cases of suspected portal biliopathy.
- ✗ Venous collaterals on the surface of the liver can be a bleeding risk if procedures are attempted.
- ✗ Portal venous occlusion can change hepatic perfusion and limit detection of hepatic lesions on cross-sectional imaging studies.

Case 92

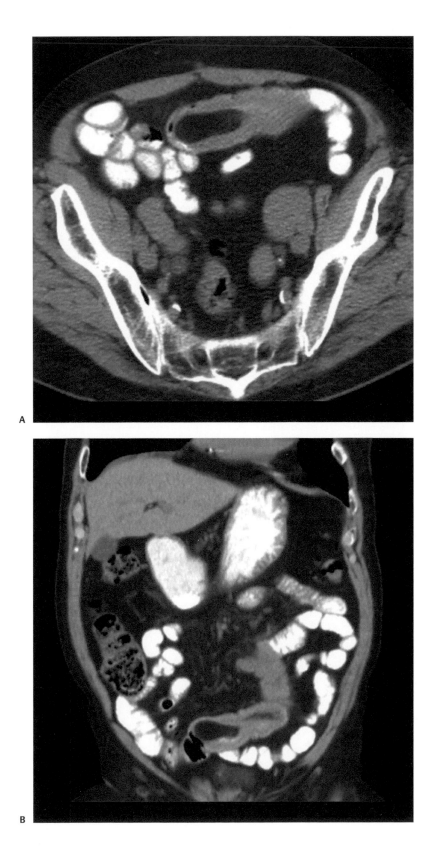

■ Clinical Presentation

A 75-year-old male presents with abdominal pain.

■ Imaging Findings

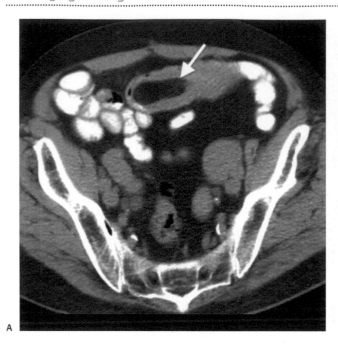 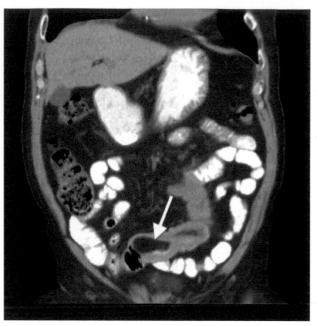

(A) Axial computed tomography (CT) shows a fatty mass in the small bowel (*arrow*). **(B)** Coronal CT shows the fatty mass as a lead point for an intussusception (*arrow*).

■ Differential Diagnosis

- ***Small bowel intussusception with lipoma as a lead point.***

■ Essential Facts

- Intussusception is classified based on location: enteroenteric, ileocolic, ileocecal, or colocolic.
- Intussusception can occur with or without a lead point.
- Non–leadpoint intussusception tends to be transient without bowel wall edema and may be asymptomatic.
- Leadpoint intussusception can cause bowel wall edema and engorged vessels.
- CT appearance is a target-like mass with a cross-sectional diameter greater than that of the normal bowel.
- Benign leadpoint lesions include lipoma, leiomyoma, hemangioma, and neurofibroma. Lipoma is the most common benign cause of colocolic intussusception in adults.
- Malignant leadpoint lesions include metastasis, adenocarcinoma, and lymphadenopathy from malignant causes.

■ Other Imaging Findings

- Ultrasound is useful to detect intussusception in children; the telescoping bowel has a target appearance.

✓ Pearls and ✗ Pitfalls

- ✓ The classic target appearance helps detect the site of intussusception.
- ✓ Bowel wall edema and bowel obstruction are indications that the intussusception is severe and may need intervention.
- ✗ Small masses may be missed as a leadpoint.
- ✗ Lipomatosis of the ileocecal valve can mimic an intussusception.

Case 93

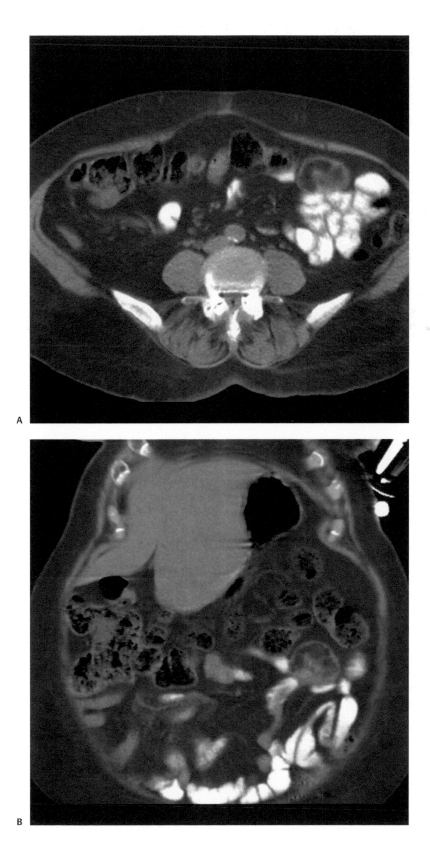

■ Clinical Presentation

A 54-year-old male with history of recent surgery presents with abdominal pain.

■ Imaging Findings

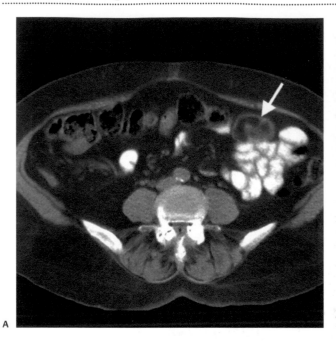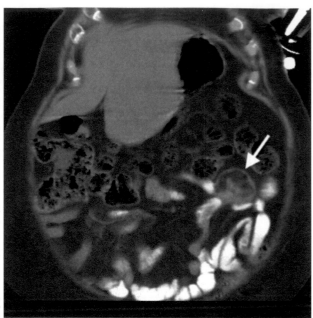

A   B

(A) Axial computed tomography (CT) shows a wall-demarcated mass in the left abdomen with fatty components adherent to the parietal peritoneum and abutting the bowel (*arrow*). (B) Coronal CT shows the fatty mass with internal fat stranding (*arrow*). Adjacent bowel is normal.

■ Differential Diagnosis

- **Omental infarction:** Infarction of a portion of the omentum.
- *Epiploic appendagitis:* Torsion and infarction of the colonic epiploic appendages.

■ Essential Facts

- Omental infarction is more common in the right abdomen due to the greater length and mobility of the omentum on that side.
- CT shows a primary fatty, encapsulated mass with soft tissue stranding adherent to the parietal peritoneum.
- Primary omental torsion describes a mobile segment of the omentum that rotates around a proximal fixed point in the absence of any associated intra-abdominal pathology. This entity is more common in the right lower quadrant.
- Secondary omental torsion occurs as a result of surgery or a traumatic injury and is located near the surgical or pathological site.

■ Other Imaging Findings

- Ultrasound can detect omental infarction as an ovoid area of avascular echogenic fat at the site of point tenderness.

✓ Pearls and ✗ Pitfalls

- ✓ Acute appendicitis and diverticulitis also cause fat stranding: a thorough evaluation is warranted to exclude other causes of this finding.
- ✓ Omental infarctions can be the cause of postoperative pain.
- ✗ Omental infarctions should not be mistaken for the very rare omental liposarcoma, which is space-occupying and increases in size over time.
- ✗ Omental metastasis with nodular, dense changes and thickening of the omentum can mimic omental infarction.

Case 94

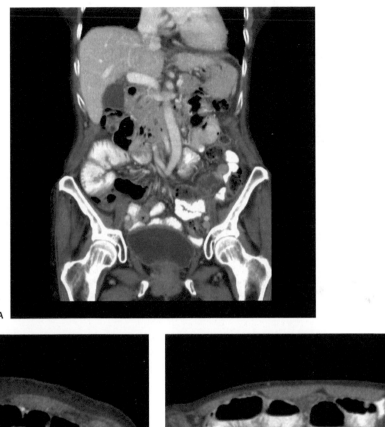

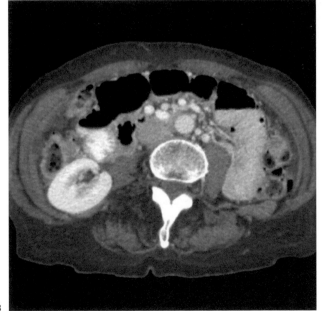

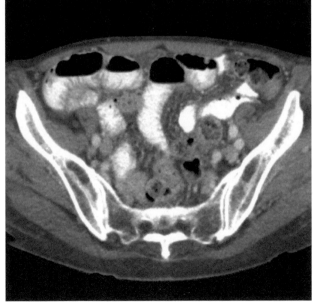

■ Clinical Presentation

A 76-year-old female with weight loss, abdominal pain, and bloating.

■ Imaging Findings

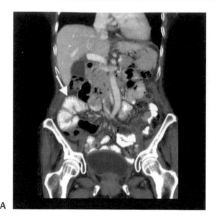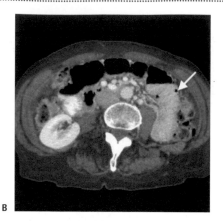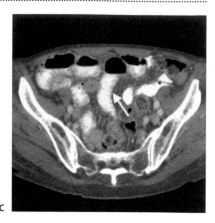

A   B   C

(A) Coronal contrast-enhanced computed tomography (CT) shows ileal fold thickening and bland appearing jejunal folds (*arrow*). **(B)** Axial contrast-enhanced CT shows the featureless dilated jejunal loops in the upper abdomen (*arrow*). **(C)** Axial contrast-enhanced CT shows the ileal loops with a jejunal type fold pattern (*arrow*).

■ Differential Diagnosis

- *Celiac disease:* Chronic autoimmune disorder induced after ingestion of gluten proteins that results in progressive small bowel villus inflammation.
- *Inflammatory bowel disease:* Chronic autoimmune disease that affects the gastrointestinal tract and can result in villous atrophy.

■ Essential Facts

- Celiac disease is an autoimmune disorder that results in progressive degrees of villus inflammation with resulting induction of crypt hyperplasia.
- Contrast findings in the small bowel are dilution, dilatation, slow transit, flocculation, and laminar flow.
- There is reversal of the jejunal-ileal fold pattern with a bland jejunal wall with or without wall thickening.
- Transient small bowel intussusception.
- Enlarged mesenteric nodes.

■ Other Imaging Findings

- On magnetic resonance imaging, coronal single shot fast spin echo sequences can be used to compare the fold pattern, which is similar to that seen on CT.

✓ Pearls and ✗ Pitfalls

✓ Compare the jejunal folds and the ileal folds on the coronal plane.
✓ Positive oral contrast shows the contrast distribution in the bowel, whereas neutral oral contrast agents only show the fold pattern.
✗ Laminar oral contrast flow in the bowel lumen can mimic intussusception.
✗ Dilated loops of bowel should not be mistaken for ileus or obstruction.

Case 95

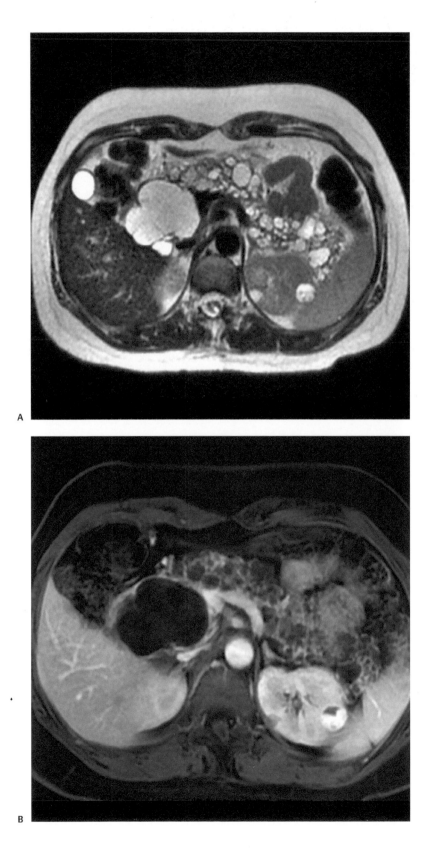

A

B

■ Clinical Presentation

A 35-year-old man with abnormal abdominal ultrasound seen for further evaluation.

■ Imaging Findings

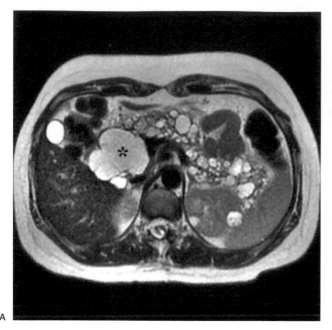
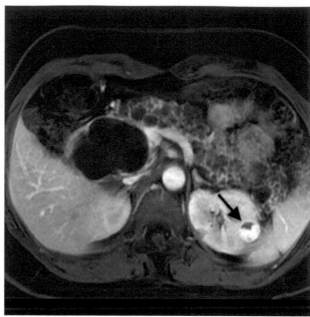

(A) Axial T2-weighted imaging shows a dominant cyst in the pancreatic head and innumerable cysts replacing the pancreatic parenchyma (*asterisk*). Note the cystic lesion in left kidney. (B) Axial fast spoiled gradient echo +C shows enhancing left renal mass (*arrow*).

■ Differential Diagnosis

• **Von Hippel Lindau (VHL) syndrome:** Rare autosomal dominant disease with high penetrance with development of benign and malignant tumors.

■ Essential Facts

• Multiorgan involvement.
• Renal cysts (59–63%) and renal cell carcinomas (25–45%) in the kidney.
• Pancreatic lesions consist of pancreatic cysts (50–91%), serous microcystic adenomas (12%), pancreas neuroendocrine tumors (5–17%), and rarely adenocarcinomas.
• Pheochromocytomas (0–60%).

■ Other Imaging Findings

• Ultrasound is a good modality to evaluate the renal lesions for growth. Computed tomography is also excellent for evaluating the pancreas and kidneys but adds a radiation risk. Patients with VHL syndrome have to undergo annual screening for renal and pancreatic masses.

✓ Pearls and ✗ Pitfalls

✓ Presence of pancreatic cysts and renal cysts should prompt genetic screening.
✓ Renal cell carcinomas and pancreatic neuroendocrine tumors are generally slow growing.
✗ The innumerable pancreatic cysts can limit evaluation for solid neoplasms.
✗ Small adrenal and extra-adrenal pheochromocytomas can be difficult to detect.

Case 96

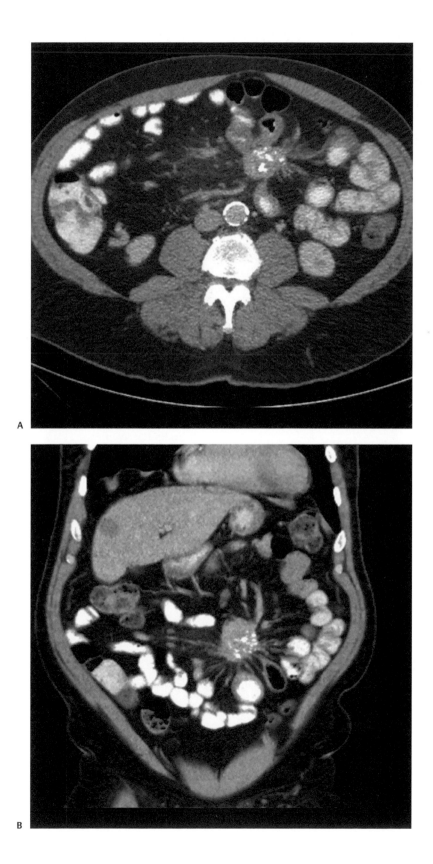

■ Clinical Presentation

A 64-year-old male presents with abdominal pain.

■ **Imaging Findings**

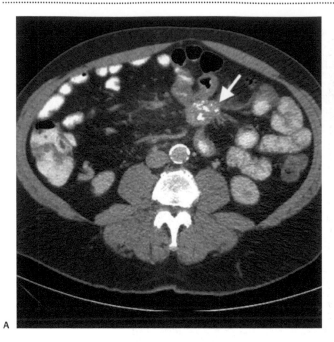 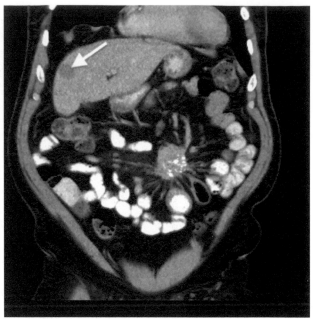

A   B

(A) Axial contrast-enhanced computed tomography (CT) shows a solid, spiculated mass in the mesentery with calcifications (*arrow*). Note the bowel kinking, tethering, and angulation. **(B)** Coronal contrast-enhanced CT shows the tethering of bowel loops and metastatic disease in the liver (*arrow*).

■ **Differential Diagnosis**

• ***Carcinoid:*** A tumor of neuroendocrine origin that can arise from the gastrointestinal tract.
• *Sclerosing mesenteritis:* Benign entity manifested by fat necrosis, inflammation, fibrosis, and mesenteric retraction.
• *Treated lymphoma:* Mesenteric lymph nodes undergoing treatment can calcify and undergo fibrosis.

■ **Essential Facts**

• Carcinoid describes a heterogeneous group of neuroendocrine tumors with a spectrum ranging from benign and indolent to aggressive and metastatic.
• Mesenteric carcinoids are usually metastatic from a primary in the small bowel (40–80% of cases). A primary mesenteric carcinoid is rare.
• Tumors secrete serotonin that incites a local desmoplastic reaction, which on multidetector CT gives a characteristic appearance of bowel kinking, tethering, angulation, and, at times, obstruction.
• Calcification is seen in 70% of mesenteric masses with three patterns described: small stippled, coarse dense, and diffuse.

• Tumors show arterial enhancement and delayed washout.
• Mesenteric lesions can cause arterial and venous narrowing and occlusion.

■ **Other Imaging Findings**

• Magnetic resonance enterography with multiphasic contrast sequences is useful in detection and staging. The lesions are hypointense on T1-weighted images, heterogeneously hyperintense on T2-weighted images, and show heterogeneous enhancement.

✓ **Pearls and ✗ Pitfalls**

✓ A good arterial phase study about 30 seconds after iodinated contrast injection helps detect small carcinoids.
✓ Coronal multiplanar reformation helps identify small masses; the primary tumor is usually notably smaller than the nodal metastasis.
✗ Small bowel carcinoid tumors may show only an area of bowel wall thickening.
✗ Carcinoid tumors can be multifocal, necessitating a dedicated search pattern.

Case 97

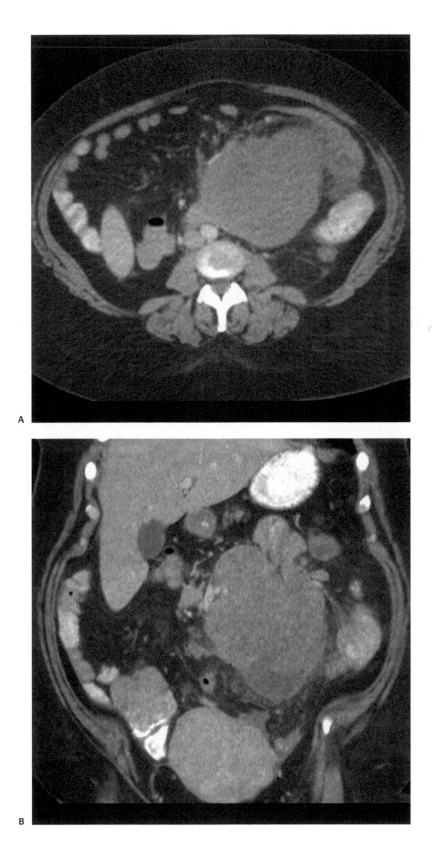

A 53-year-old female with abdominal pain, fullness, and a palpable abdominal mass.

■ **Imaging Findings**

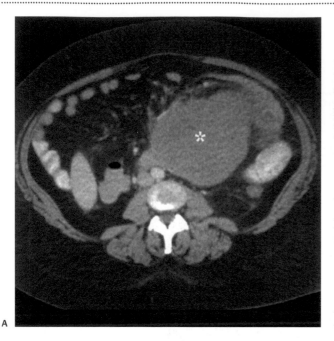
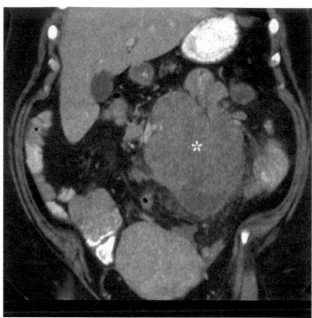

A   B

(A) Axial contrast-enhanced computed tomography (CT) shows a soft tissue mass in the mesentery with midlevel enhancement and no areas of necrosis (*asterisk*). **(B)** Coronal contrast-enhanced CT shows the mass involving loops of bowel in the left upper abdomen (*asterisk*).

■ **Differential Diagnosis**

• ***Mesenteric desmoid fibromatosis:*** Benign locally aggressive desmoid tumor.
• *Lymphoma:* B-cell lymphoma can involve the mesenteric lymph nodes and the small bowel.
• *Gastrointestinal stromal tumor (GIST):* Mesenchymal neoplasms arising from smooth muscle interstitial cells.

■ **Essential Facts**

• Mesenteric desmoid fibromatosis is a locally aggressive fibroblastic neoplasm.
• It may occur in isolation or in association with the hereditary syndrome called familial adenomatous polyposis (FAP).
• Masses show mild to moderate enhancement. Necrosis and calcifications are extremely rare.
• Imaging features are a soft tissue mass with radiating spicules extending into the adjacent mesenteric fat.

• Abdominal wall is the most common site of disease.
• Bone involvement can be present in 5–30% of tumors.
• Locally recurrent after resection.

■ **Other Imaging Findings**

• On magnetic resonance imaging, desmoid fibromatosis is T1-hypointense to muscle and is variable on T2 imaging with some tumors appearing hypointense.

✓ **Pearls and ✗ Pitfalls**

✓ Has a smooth border with thin spicules that infiltrate the fat.
✓ In FAP, it is associated with prior surgery.
✗ May be indistinguishable from malignant mesenteric masses.
✗ Cystic degeneration suggests a malignant entity such as GIST.

Case 98

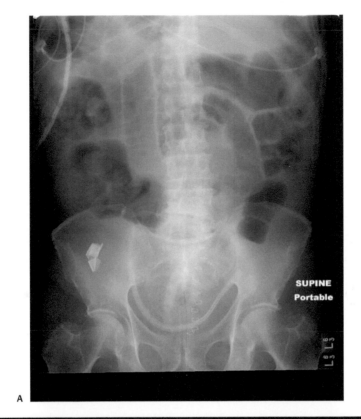

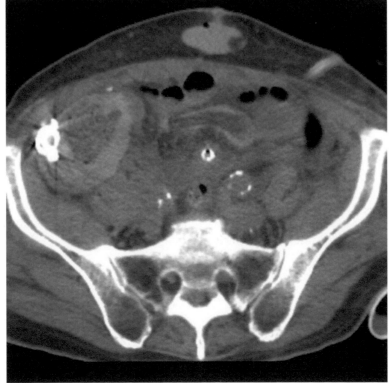

■ **Clinical Presentation**

A 97-year-old male with abdominal pain.

■ Imaging Findings

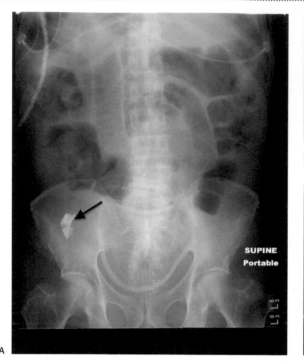
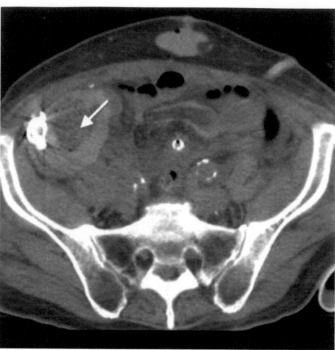

(A) Plain film radiograph shows the radiopaque marker of a laparotomy sponge in the right lower quadrant (*arrow*). (B) Computed tomography (CT) shows a mass in the right lower abdomen with a radiopaque object within it (*arrow*).

■ Differential Diagnosis

- ***Retained surgical laparotomy sponge (gossypiboma):*** Retained foreign body that causes a chronic abscess and inflammation.
- *Abdominal abscess:* Pus collection in the abdomen.

■ Essential Facts

- Surgical sponges have different types of radiopaque markers to identify them on radiography.
- Routine postoperative radiographs after surgery reduce the risk of a retained foreign body.
- Fistulization between organs may occur.
- Presents as an abdominal mass with internal bubbles and a thick wall with peripheral enhancement.

■ Other Imaging Findings

- Magnetic resonance imaging can be used to detect a gossypiboma, which appears as a soft tissue mass with a whorled internal configuration and thick peripheral enhancement.

✓ Pearls and ✗ Pitfalls

✓ Radiographs are a quick and easy way to detect a retained sponge using the radiopaque marker.
✓ Evaluate for complications such as abscess or fistulae.
✗ The mass may be mistaken for a malignancy or abscess.
✗ Streak artifact from the radiopaque marker can obscure anatomy on CT.

Case 99

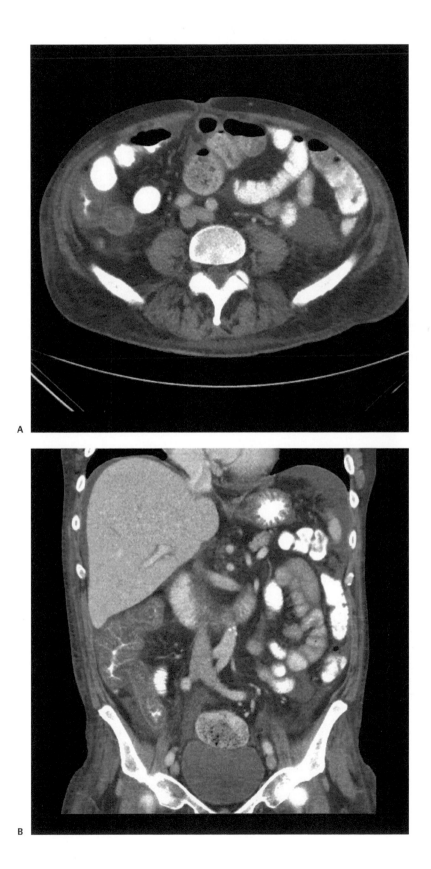

A

B

■ Clinical Presentation

A 55-year-old male presents with history of acute myeloid leukemia and chemotherapy with neutropenia and abdominal pain.

■ Imaging Findings

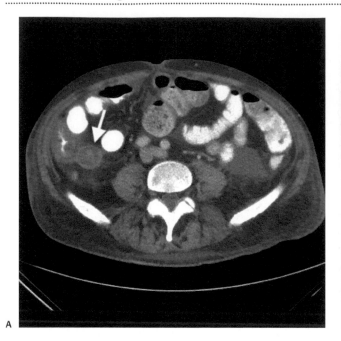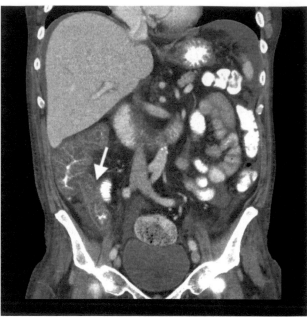

A   B

(A) Axial contrast-enhanced computed tomography (CT) shows diffuse thickening of the terminal ileum and the cecum (*arrow*). (B) Coronal contrast-enhanced CT shows inflammation and fat stranding around the terminal ileum and cecum (*arrow*).

■ Differential Diagnosis

- **Neutropenic enterocolitis (typhlitis):** A severe condition affecting immunocompromised patients manifested by intestinal edema, engorged vessels, and a disrupted mucosal surface.
- *Inflammatory bowel disease:* A chronic inflammatory condition of the colon and/or small bowel.
- *Infectious ileocolitis:* Infection of the small bowel and/or colon.
- *Ischemic ileocolitis:* Caused by a vascular insult to the small bowel or colon.

■ Essential Facts

- Neutropenic enterocolitis, or typhlitis, occurs in immunocompromised patients; certain chemotherapeutic drugs can cause direct mucosal injury and ulceration.
- Incidence is ~5.6% of hospitalized patients with hematologic malignancies.
- Mortality can be as high as 50%.

- CT is excellent in diagnosing neutropenic enterocolitis. Imaging features include colonic mural thickening, low-density areas representing edema and/or necrosis, pericolic inflammation, ascites, pneumatosis intestinalis, and, in severe cases, free air indicating perforation.
- Small bowel is involved in 66% of cases.

■ Other Imaging Findings

- Magnetic resonance imaging shows thick edematous small bowel and colon segment with hyperenhancement of the mucosa.

✓ Pearls and ✗ Pitfalls

✓ Intravenous contrast is recommended to evaluate mucosal enhancement.
✓ Right colon is most commonly involved.
✗ Mimics include *Clostridium difficile* pseudomembranous colitis.
✗ May involve a short segment of small bowel.

Case 100

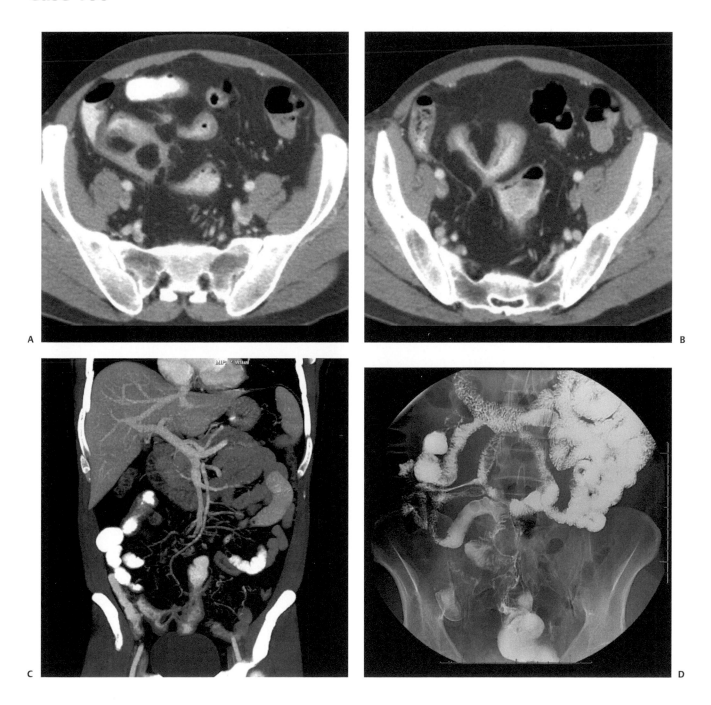

A

B

C

D

■ **Clinical Presentation**

A 45-year-old male presents with abdominal pain and weight loss.

■ Imaging Findings

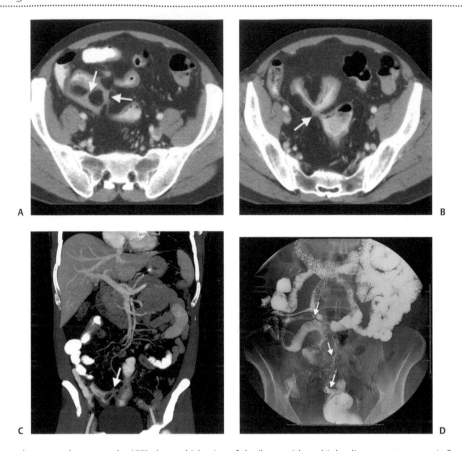

(A) Axial contrast-enhanced computed tomography (CT) shows thickening of the ileum with multiple, discrete enteroenteric fistulae (*arrows*). Note the fibrofatty proliferation. **(B)** Axial contrast-enhanced CT shows an angulated loop of ileum with a connection to the colon forming an enterocolic fistula (*arrow*). **(C)** Coronal maximum intensity projection contrast-enhanced CT shows the extensive ileal and colonic fistulae (*arrow*). **(D)** Barium small bowel follow-through shows the extensive network of enteroenteric and enterocolic fistulae (*arrows*). Note the contrast in the rectum but no contrast in the descending colon.

■ Differential Diagnosis

• ***Fistulizing Crohn's disease:*** An inflammatory bowel disease that causes transmural inflammation resulting in fistulae, abscesses, and fissures.

■ Essential Facts

• In Crohn's disease, the small intestine is involved in 80% of cases, most commonly at the terminal ileum.
• The colon is affected either with (50% of cases) or without (15–20%) involvement of the small intestine.
• Imaging can show fistulae, abscesses, fibrofatty proliferation, increased vascularity of the vasa recta, and mesenteric lymphadenopathy.

■ Other Imaging Findings

• Magnetic resonance (MR) enterography is an excellent modality to evaluate the small bowel for active inflammation and is the modality of choice for perianal fistulae.
• Barium small bowel follow-through can show areas of bowel involvement, fistulae, strictures, and adhesions. The small bowel follow-through facilitates evaluation of bowel peristalsis.

✓ Pearls and ✗ Pitfalls

✓ Use a negative oral contrast agent such as VoLumen (Bracco Diagnostics Inc.) to evaluate the small bowel mucosa.
✓ Look for skip lesions throughout the gastrointestinal tract.
✗ CT with positive oral contrast can miss mucosal inflammation as it obscures the enhancing mucosa.
✗ Collapsed loops of bowel can limit evaluation and mimic bowel wall thickening.

Case Questions and Answers

The questions and answers in the following section are numbered as cases 1 through 100. The questions correspond to the respectively numbered case reviews and are intended to be answered after working through the cases.

■ Case 1

1. The reason for HCC enhancement at the arterial phase is because:
   a) HCC has a predominately hepatic portal venous blood supply
   b) HCC has a predominately hepatic arterial blood supply
   c) HCC has well-developed lymphatics
   d) HCC causes venous occlusion

   The correct answer is (**b**). HCC typically has a predominately arterial blood supply that causes its avid arterial enhancement in relation to background liver.

2. A newly detected liver lesion by ultrasound in a cirrhotic patient that measures over 1 cm requires:
   a) Single phase CT with contrast
   b) Biopsy
   c) Four-phase CT with contrast
   d) Repeat ultrasound in 3 months

   The correct answer is (**c**). A new or growing liver nodule in a cirrhotic liver requires a four-phase CT with contrast for characterization.

■ Case 2

1. The best phase of imaging the liver by CT for breast cancer metastasis is:
   a) Non-contrast phase CT
   b) Arterial phase CT
   c) Portal venous phase CT
   d) Delayed phase CT

   The correct answer is (**c**). Breast cancer is best imaged on portal venous phase as hypodense metastatic lesions because breast cancer metastases are mostly hypovascular in relation to the liver.

2. Which of the following entity does not produce a nodular hepatic appearance?
   a) Treated liver metastasis
   b) Hepatic venous thrombosis
   c) Chronic portal venous thrombosis
   d) Fat deposition in the liver

   The correct answer is (**d**). Fat deposition in the liver manifests as hepatomegaly with a smooth contour.

■ Case 3

1. The preferred treatment for hepatic abscess > 5 cm is:
   a) Percutaneous needle drainage
   b) Percutaneous catheter drainage
   c) Surgical drainage
   d) Antibiotics

   The correct answer is (**b**). Percutaneous placed catheter drainage is the preferred method of treatment of solitary hepatic abscess > 5 cm. Needle drainage is used for lesions < 5 cm whereas the surgical approach is used for multiple abscess, complicated abscess, or inadequate response to percutaneous drainage.

2. The most common cause of pyogenic liver abscess is:
   a) Gastrointestinal source
   b) Biliary source
   c) Hematologic source
   d) Trauma

   Correct answer is (**b**). Infectious diseases of the biliary tract are the most common cause of hepatic abscess.

■ Case 4

1. Portal vein occlusion in the setting of a mass-forming cholangiocarcinoma is likely due to:
   a) Benign external compression
   b) Malignant invasion of the portal vein
   c) Thrombosis due to hypercoagulable state
   d) Portal hypertension

   The correct answer is (**b**). Portal venous thrombosis at or near the lesion must be considered malignant as the portal system forms an important route of spread of the disease.

2. The value of the delayed phase CT (3 to 30 minutes) in imaging suspected cholangiocarcinoma is to:
   a) Evaluate portal venous occlusion
   b) Evaluate capsular retraction
   c) Identify satellite lesions
   d) Help characterize the lesion

   Correct answer is (**d**). Cholangiocarcinoma commonly shows delayed hyperattenuation compared to the liver due to its fibrous component, a feature that can be an important finding in characterizing the lesion.

■ Case 5

1. Which of the following lesions do not contain intralesional fat?
    a) Focal nodular hyperplasia
    b) Hepatic adenoma
    c) Hepatic angiomyolipoma
    d) Hepatic metastasis

The correct answer is (**d**). Hepatic metastases do not contain intralesional fat.

2. Focal nodular hyperplasia does not contain which of the following:
    a) Hepatic arterial supply
    b) Hepatic venous drainage
    c) Well-formed biliary drainage
    d) Central scar

The correct answer is (**c**). Focal nodular hyperplasia lacks well-formed biliary drainage. This is responsible for the accumulation of hepatobiliary contrast agents within the lesion.

■ Case 6

1. Focal fatty infiltration can be differentiated from FFS by which of the following findings:
    a) Signal loss on T1-FSPGR in-phase
    b) Signal gain on T1-FSPGR in-phase
    c) Signal loss on T1-FSPGR opposed-phase imaging
    d) Signal gain on T1-FSPGR opposed-phase imaging

The correct answer is (**c**). Focal fatty infiltration shows signal loss on T1-FSPGR opposed-phase imaging.

2. Which of the following is *not* characteristic of FFS?
    a) Mass effect on adjacent vessels
    b) Differences in perfusion on arterial phase imaging
    c) Location near the portal vein
    d) Signal loss on T1-FSPGR opposed-phase imaging

The correct answer is (**a**). FFS does not have regional mass effect since it consists of normal liver parenchyma.

■ Case 7

1. Which of the following lesions is hypointense on T1-weighted imaging?
    a) Melanoma metastasis
    b) Hepatic cyst
    c) Adenoma with hemorrhage
    d) Hepatocellular carcinoma

The correct answer is (**b**). Hepatic cysts are typically hypointense on T1-weighted imaging. The remainder of the lesions can be T1-hyperintense due to varying amounts of hemorrhage or protein.

2. T1-FSPGR fat-suppressed postcontrast images with subtraction are useful in which of the following cases:
    a) Evaluation of liver with suspected fatty infiltration
    b) Evaluation of liver with suspected hepatic cysts
    c) Evaluation of liver with suspected hemangioma
    d) Evaluation of liver with suspected inherently T1-hyperintense lesion

The correct answer is (**d**). Hepatic lesions that cause T-shortening (T1-hyperintense) can be difficult to evaluate for enhancement. The use of subtraction images obtained by postprocessing by subtracting the precontrast images from the postcontrast images allows one to evaluate the lesion of "true" enhancement.

■ Case 8

1. The most common cause of concurrent hypodense hepatic and splenic lesions in an immunocompromised patient is:
    a) Metastasis
    b) Sarcoid
    c) Amyloid
    d) Disseminated infection with microabscesses

The correct answer is (**d**). In an immunocompromised patient, an infectious etiology, in particular disseminated fungal microabscesses, should be the leading diagnosis. If there is associated low-density lymphadenopathy, infectious tuberculosis should be considered.

2. Which of the following infections are most likely to evolve to calcinations after the acute phase:
    a) Amebic abscess
    b) Histoplasmosis
    c) Candida
    d) Sarcoid

The correct answer is (**b**). Histoplasmosis is the most common granulomatous disease in North America. The granulomatous infection incites an immune inflammatory response leading to granuloma formation. During the active phase, granulomas are imaged as nearly uniform small hypodense lesions that heal and calcify over time.

■ Case 9

1. The best modality to characterize a hepatic hemangioma is:
    a) Contrast-enhanced multiphase MRI
    b) F18–fluorodeoxyglucose positron emission tomography/CT
    c) Portal venous phase CT
    d) Ultrasound

The correct answer is (**a**). Contrast-enhanced multiphase MRI is very accurate in the diagnosis of hepatic hemangioma with a reported sensitivity and specificity of 98% and accuracy of 99%.

2. Which of the following is not characteristic of a giant cavernous hemangioma?
    a) Central fibrous scar
    b) Calcifications in the lesion
    c) Peripheral nodular discontinuous enhancement
    d) Uniform arterial enhancement

The correct answer is (**d**). Uniform arterial enhancement is characteristic of small flash-filling hemangiomas. Giant cavernous hemangiomas tend to have a slower lesion enhancement and progressive centripetal fill-in.

■ Case 10

1. Which of the following is associated with a lesion suspected as focal fat deposition?
    a) Geographic borders
    b) Mass effect
    c) Distortion in the course of vessels
    d) Arterial enhancement

The correct answer is (**a**). Focal fat deposition has geographic borders, no mass effect, and does not distort traversing vessels. The lesion usually enhances similarly to liver or slightly less than liver.

2. Which of the following imaging tests is specific for focal fat?
    a) Ultrasound
    b) Contrast-enhanced CT
    c) F18–fluorodeoxyglucose positron emission tomography
    d) Chemical-shift magnetic resonance imaging

The correct answer is (**d**). Chemical-shift magnetic resonance imaging is easily performed and is a confirmative imaging test to diagnose focal fat deposition by loss of signal on opposed-phase images in comparison with in-phase images.

■ Case 11

1. Screening is done in patients with nonalcoholic liver disease to detect:
    a) Hepatic adenomas
    b) Hepatocellular carcinoma
    c) Hepatic metastasis
    d) Cholangiocarcinoma

The correct answer is (**b**). Patients with nonalcoholic liver disease have increased risk of developing hepatocellular carcinoma, and screening is performed in at-risk patients.

2. The MRI sequence used to quantify hepatic steatosis is:
    a) In/opposed phase imaging
    b) 2-point Dixon technique
    c) T1-FSPGR with and without fat saturation
    d) Iterative decomposition of water and fat with echo asymmetry and the least-squares estimation

The correct answer is (**d**). IDEAL imaging is used to quantify hepatic fatty infiltration. As it is able to separate water and fat, it is also used for robust fat saturation.

■ Case 12

1. Biliary hamartomas result from developmental malformations of the:
    a) Tectal plate
    b) Basal plate
    c) Ductal plate
    d) Biliary plate

The correct answer is (**c**). Biliary hamartomas are developmental malformations of the ductal plate, which cause partial or complete arrest of the processes involved in the development of the intrahepatic bile ducts.

2. Biliary hamartomas are different from the biliary dilation seen in Caroli's disease and syndrome as they:
    a) Do not communicate with the biliary tree
    b) Accumulate hepatobiliary agent on delayed imaging
    c) Can be diagnosed with a retrograde cholangiogram
    d) Have no added risk for cholangiocarcinoma

The correct answer is (**a**). Biliary hamartomas do not communicate with the biliary tree.

Case 13

1. Which of the following is needed to diagnose a fat-deficient HAML?
   a) Lesion biopsy
   b) History of tuberous sclerosis complex
   c) Multiphasic magnetic resonance imaging of the liver
   d) Multiphasic CT of the liver

The correct answer is (**a**). HAML are diagnosed by their macroscopic fat. In its absence, the lesion may need to be biopsied to establish the diagnosis.

2. HAML are lesions of which cell line?
   a) Epithelial origin
   b) Mesenchymal origin
   c) Epithelioid origin
   d) Sarcomatoid origin

The correct answer is (**b**). HAML are benign mesenchymal tumors.

Case 14

1. Which of the following is a characteristic of primary hepatic lymphoma?
   a) Splenic involvement
   b) Osseous involvement
   c) Hepatic involvement
   d) Mediastinal involvement

The correct answer is (**c**). Primary hepatic lymphoma is a disease that is confined to the liver and perihepatic nodal sites at patient presentation, without other distant organ involvement.

2. Specific imaging features of hepatic lymphoma include:
   a) Arterial enhancement
   b) Portal venous washout
   c) Delayed imaging washout
   d) No specific imaging features

The correct answer is (**d**). Lymphoma in the liver typically is hypoenhancing to liver, which is not specific. Biopsy may be necessary for a diagnosis. The use of multiphasic CT is not always useful.

Case 15

1. Budd-Chiari syndrome is primarily due to:
   a) Portal venous occlusion
   b) Hepatic artery occlusion
   c) Hepatic venous occlusion
   d) Hepatic fibrosis

The correct answer is (**c**). Budd-Chiari syndrome is due to hepatic venous outflow occlusion.

2. In acute Budd-Chiari syndrome, which of the following can be seen?
   a) Hypoattenuating hepatic veins
   b) Caudate hypertrophy
   c) Hepatocellular carcinoma
   d) Calcification of the inferior vena cava

The correct answer is (**a**). Hypoattenuating hepatic veins, splenomegaly, and ascites can been seen in the acute phase.

Case 16

1. The measurement that includes lesion attenuation to evaluate response in gastrointestinal stromal tumors is:
   a) Choi criteria
   b) Resist 1.0
   c) Resist 1.1
   d) mResist

The correct answer is (**a**). Choi criteria take into account lesion attenuation in assessing disease progression.

2. Which of these is a common metastatic disease site for gastrointestinal stromal tumor?
   a) Lung
   b) Peritoneum
   c) Spleen
   d) Bone

The correct answer is (**b**). Another common site of metastasis apart from the liver is the peritoneum.

Case 17

1. Which is the most common subtype of HCC?
   a) Hepatocyte-nuclear-factor-1α mutated type
   b) β-catenin-mutated type with upregulation of glutamine synthetase
   c) Inflammatory type with serum-amyloid-A overexpression
   d) Unclassified hepatocellular adenoma

The correct answer is (**c**). The inflammatory type with serum-amyloid-A overexpression is the most common subtype accounting for about 45–55% of lesions. They were initially described as telangiectatic focal nodular hyperplasia, characterized by inflammatory infiltrates and frequent sinusoidal dilatation.

2. Which of the following subtype of HCC contains fat?
   a) Hepatocyte-nuclear-factor-1α mutated type
   b) β-catenin-mutated type with upregulation of glutamine synthetase
   c) Inflammatory type with serum-amyloid-A overexpression
   d) Unclassified hepatocellular adenoma

The correct answer is (**a**). The hepatocyte-nuclear-factor-1α mutated have a predominant intralesional fat component.

▪ Case 18

1. Biliary cystadenoma most commonly arises from:
   a) The intrahepatic biliary tree
   b) The extrahepatic biliary tree
   c) The peritoneum
   d) The retroperitoneum

The correct answer is (**a**). Biliary cystadenoma tends to arise from the intrahepatic biliary tree and presents as a cystic hepatic mass.

2. Treatment for biliary cystadenoma is:
   a) Ablation
   b) Surgical excision
   c) Aspiration
   d) Follow-up imaging

The correct answer is (**b**). Surgical excision of the lesion is the treatment of choice. Lesions with cyst complexity can be difficult to differentiate from the malignant form.

▪ Case 19

1. PSC is characterized by:
   a) Intrahepatic biliary strictures
   b) Extrahepatic biliary strictures
   c) Both intra- and extrahepatic biliary strictures
   d) Peribiliary cysts

The correct answer is (**c**). PSC affects both the intrahepatic and extrahepatic biliary tree and can cause strictures of varying degrees and lengths.

2. The concern in the development of a new of dominant stricture is:
   a) The development of malignant cholangiocarcinoma
   b) Focal biliary inflammation
   c) Biliary lithiasis
   d) Development of biliary ischemia

The correct answer is (**a**). The primary concern in screening patients is the early detection of cholangiocarcinoma, which can manifest as a new or dominant stricture.

▪ Case 20

1. Which of the following is considered extrahepatic spread?
   a) Metastatic disease in the liver
   b) Invasion through the gallbladder fossa
   c) Portal tract invasion
   d) Omental disease

The correct answer is (**d**). Omental disease is considered extrahepatic disease spread. Direct hepatic invasion and portal tract invasion are modes of hepatic spread from resectable gallbladder carcinoma.

2. The most common imaging presentation of gallbladder carcinoma is:
   a) A mass replacing the lumen of the gallbladder
   b) Focal asymmetric wall thickening
   c) Polypoid mass
   d) Exophytic mass

The correct answer is (**a**). Mass occupying or replacing the gallbladder lumen accounts for 40 to 65% of cases at initial presentation.

▪ Case 21

1. A specific sign of gangrenous cholecystitis is:
   a) Pericholecystic fluid
   b) Distended gallbladder
   c) Thick gallbladder wall
   d) Intraluminal membranes

The correct answer is (**d**). Intraluminal membranes are a specific sign of gangrenous cholecystitis. It indicates sloughing of necrotic membranes into the lumen of the gallbladder. Other specific signs include gas in the wall or lumen, adjacent abscess, and an absent or irregular wall.

2. The emergent treatment for gangrenous cholecystitis is:
   a) Percutaneous cholecystostomy
   b) Antibiotic therapy
   c) Surgical cholecystectomy
   d) Endoscopic drainage

The correct answer is (**a**). Percutaneous cholecystostomy is an effective therapy in the acute phase of the disease when combined with antibiotics. It can serve as an effective bridge to surgery in the very ill patient. Percutaneous cholecystostomy has relatively low mortality and high technical and clinical success rates of over 90%. It can be performed at bedside using ultrasound in unstable patients. Transhepatic (most common) and transabdominal routes are used.

■ Case 22

1. The most common presentation of gallbladder adenomyomatosis is:
    a) Localized
    b) Segmental
    c) Annular
    d) Diffuse

The correct answer is (**a**). Localized form of gallbladder adenomyomatosis is the most common presentation and occurs at the fundus of the gallbladder.

2. The most important feature on CT and MRI in differentiating gallbladder adenomyomatosis from carcinoma is:
    a) Fundal location
    b) Nodular enhancement
    c) No invasive features
    d) Cystic-appearing spaces in the mass

The correct answer is (**d**). On MRI and CT, cystic-appearing spaces represent the most specific feature to detect gallbladder adenomyomatosis. The remaining features can be seen with either entity.

■ Case 23

1. The treatment of choice for symptomatic choledocholithiasis is:
    a) Surgical exploration
    b) Endoscopic retrograde cholangiopancreatography with stone removal and drainage
    c) Percutaneous biliary drainage
    d) Lithotripsy

The correct answer is (**b**). Endoscopic retrograde cholangiopancreatography and drainage is the treatment of choice as they are minimally invasive and can facilitate balloon-assisted stone removal and stent placement if needed.

2. Compared to CT, MRCP:
    a) Can detect noncalcified stones
    b) Is noninvasive
    c) Is quicker to perform
    d) Cannot image the intrahepatic biliary tree

The correct answer is (**a**). MRCP detects noncalcified stones that CT may miss. All sizable stones of different compositions appear as filling defects on the T2-weighted MRCP sequences. Bile pigment stones can be T1-hyperintense on three-dimensional fast spoiled gradient echo imaging.

■ Case 24

1. Mirizzi's syndrome is caused by an impacted stone in which of the following locations:
    a) Common hepatic duct
    b) Common bile duct
    c) Cystic duct
    d) Pancreatic duct

The correct answer is (**c**). Mirizzi's syndrome is caused by impacted stone in the cystic duct or gallbladder neck causing common hepatic duct obstruction.

2. The major risk in either open or laparoscopic treatment is:
    a) Abscess
    b) Incomplete biliary decompression
    c) Dropped gallstone
    d) Biliary injury

The correct answer is (**d**). Biliary injury during surgery is the major risk in surgical therapy as direct visualization can be difficult because significant inflammation in the region causes obliteration of the fat.

■ Case 25

1. Which of the following modalities is the best at depicting the communication between the biliary tree and the biloma?
    a) ERCP
    b) Computed tomography
    c) Ultrasonography
    d) Hepatobiliary cholescintigraphy

The correct answer is (**a**). ERCP is excellent at depicting the site of communication of the biliary system with the biloma. Other modalities can demonstrate the collection, but the site of leak may not be evident.

2. The best management of biloma is by:
    a) Surgical washout
    b) ERCP
    c) Percutaneous drainage
    d) Biliary stenting

The correct answer is (**c**). Image-guided percutaneous drainage is excellent for draining bilomas. In addition, bile duct injury can be managed with percutaneous transhepatic biliary drain placement to divert bile away from site of ductal injury.

■ Case 26

1. The Todani types of choledochal cysts most associated
   with malignant degeneration are:
   a) Types II and V
   b) Types II and III
   c) Types III and V
   d) Types I and IV

The correct answer is (d). Todani type I and IV cysts are
most associated with cholangiocarcinoma. Gallbladder
carcinoma is also associated with choledochal cysts.

2. Which of the following is associated with the
   development of choledochal cysts?
   a) Stenosis at the ampulla
   b) Anomalous union of the pancreatic and bile ducts
   c) Pancreatic divisum
   d) Gallbladder duplication

The correct answer is (b). Anomalous union of the pancreatic and bile ducts with the fusion occurring outside
the duodenal wall is associated with the development of
choledochal cysts.

■ Case 27

1. The most common site for dropped gallstones is:
   a) Perihepatic area
   b) Pelvis
   c) Lesser sac
   d) Greater omentum

The correct answer is (a). The most common sites for
dropped gallstones are the gallbladder fossa and Morrison's pouch.

2. The definitive treatment for symptomatic dropped
   gallstones is:
   a) Antibiotics
   b) Percutaneous drainage
   c) Imaging surveillance
   d) Surgical removal

The correct answer is (d). The treatment of symptomatic
dropped gallstones is surgical removal. All other methods
do not treat the underlying etiology for the inflammation
and infection.

■ Case 28

1. The malignancy most associated with hepatolithiasis is:
   a) Cholangiocarcinoma
   b) Gallbladder adenocarcinoma
   c) Hepatocellular carcinoma
   d) Hepatocellular adenoma

The correct answer is (a). Patients with hepatolithiasis are
at increased risk for cholangiocarcinoma caused by chronic
biliary inflammation and recurrent cholangitis.

2. The term hepatolithiasis is used to describe stones in
   the biliary tree:
   a) In the distal common bile duct
   b) In the gallbladder
   c) In the pancreatic duct
   d) In the intrahepatic bile ducts

The correct answer is (d). Hepatolithiasis is a term used to
describe stones in the biliary tree within the liver.

■ Case 29

1. The most common cause of acute bacterial cholangitis is:
   a) Malignancy
   b) Immunocompromise
   c) ERCP
   d) Choledocholithiasis

The correct answer is (d). Choledocholithiasis is the most
common cause of acute bacterial cholangitis, accounting
for 80% of cases.

2. Which of the following can occur with chronic
   bacterial cholangitis?
   a) Hepatic abscess
   b) Cholangiocarcinoma
   c) Bile peritonitis
   d) Hepatic vein thrombosis

The correct answer is (b). Chronic infection
leads to chronic inflammation, which can lead to
cholangiocarcinoma.

■ Case 30

1. Normal pancreas signal on magnetic resonance
   imaging (MRI) is:
   a) T1-hypointense to liver
   b) T1-hyperintense to liver
   c) T1-isointense to liver
   d) T1-hypointense to liver after contrast administration

The correct answer is (**b**). Normal pancreas signal is T1-hyperintense to liver due presence of acinar proteins. The intrinsic T1 signal decreases with age and in the setting of acute or chronic pancreatitis. Normal pancreas enhances briskly after contrast administration.

2. CT is superior to MRI in the detection of:
    a) Chronic pancreatitis
    b) Pancreatic pseudocyst
    c) Pancreatic necrosis
    d) Gas in a pancreatic fluid collection

The correct answer is (**d**). CT is superior at detecting gas in a pancreatic fluid collection. Gas in a necrotic collection indicates a pancreatic abscess.

■ Case 31
....

1. The most common cause of chronic pancreatitis in Western countries is:
    a) Alcohol abuse
    b) Chemotherapy
    c) Spider bites
    d) Gallstones

The correct answer is (**a**). Alcohol abuse is the most common cause of chronic pancreatitis.

2. Which location of calcifications is considered diagnostic of chronic pancreatitis?
    a) Only ductal calcifications
    b) Only parenchymal calcifications
    c) Diffuse parenchymal calcifications
    d) Coexisting parenchymal and intraductal calcifications

The correct answer is (**d**). Coexisting parenchymal and intraductal calcifications are diagnostic of chronic pancreatitis on CT. The distribution of pancreatic calcifications alters specificity as follows: parenchymal calcifications (67%), ductal calcifications (88%), and diffuse parenchymal calcifications (91%).

■ Case 32
....

1. Which of the following collections are associated with necrotizing pancreatitis?
    a) Pseudocyst
    b) Acute pancreatic fluid collection
    c) Walled-off necrosis
    d) Interstitial pancreatic fluid

The correct answer is (**c**). Walled-off necrosis is the end product of tissue necrosis after 4 weeks of pancreatic necrosis. Imaging shows a liquefied and nonliquefied collection of necrotic tissue with an encapsulated wall.

2. Which of the following is diagnostic of pancreatic necrosis?
    a) Parenchymal edema
    b) Fluid around the pancreas
    c) Heterogenous enhancement of the parenchyma
    d) Nonenhancing pancreatic parenchyma

The correct answer is (**d**). Nonenhancing pancreatic parenchyma is diagnostic of necrosis. It can be difficult to accurately delineate necrosis at times as there can be generalized heterogenous perfusion due to the inflammation.

■ Case 33
....

1. Which of the following would be a reason to drain a pancreatic pseudocyst?
    a) A 3-cm pseudocyst that is asymptomatic
    b) Gas, wall thickening, and fever in a patient with a 6-cm pseudocyst
    c) A rapidly expanding pseudocyst with hyperdense material
    d) A pancreatic fluid collection that formed a week after an acute bout of pancreatitis

The correct answer is (**b**). Infection of a pseudocyst is an indication for drainage. Small asymptomatic pseudocysts do not need to be drained. A rapidly expanding pseudocyst with hyperdense material suggests hemorrhage and may require embolization.

2. Which of the following would be most successful at percutaneous drainage?
    a) Soft tissue and fluid collection in the setting of pancreatic necrosis
    b) A 4-cm collection that enhances at the arterial phase
    c) Fluid collection with a well-formed fibrous wall that does not demonstrate communication to the pancreatic duct
    d) Fluid collection with a well-formed fibrous wall that has communication to the pancreatic duct

The correct answer is (**c**). Well-formed pseudocysts that do not communicate with the pancreatic duct and do not have stricture or stenosis of the duct do the best after drainage.

■ Case 34

1. Who is most likely to present with a serous cystadenoma?
   a) A 70-year-old man
   b) A 45-year-old female
   c) A 76-year-old female
   d) A 45-year-old man

The correct answer is (**c**). Serous cystadenomas are found more commonly in females compared to males in a ratio of 4:1. They typically occur in older age > 60 years and are considered "grandmother lesions."

2. Which of the following is a worrisome finding in a suspected serous cystadenoma of the pancreas?
   a) Thick, enhancing wall
   b) Central calcifications
   c) Unilocular cyst
   d) Enhancing fibrous septae

The correct answer is (**a**). The presence of a thick, enhancing wall in a cystic neoplasm suspected of being a serous cystadenoma warrants further work-up to differentiate it from a mucinous neoplasm.

■ Case 35

1. Which of the following has increased emphasis in the 2017 AJCC staging?
   a) Tumor size
   b) Venous involvement
   c) Local invasion
   d) Arterial involvement

The correct answer is (**a**). Tumor size is a good predictor of survival. Staging based on other criteria such as vascular involvement can be variable due to different expertise at various centers.

2. The most common enhancement pattern for pancreatic adenocarcinoma is:
   a) Arterial hyperenhancement
   b) Portal venous hyperenhancement
   c) Isoattenuating
   d) Hypoenhancing

The correct answer is (**d**). Most adenocarcinomas of the pancreas are hypoenhancing to the background normal pancreas. A total of 10% of adenocarcinomas are isoattenuating at CT and may need MRI for detection.

■ Case 36

1. Which of the following is a risk factor for malignancy?
   a) Size < 2 cm
   b) Connection to the main branch
   c) Thin wall
   d) Dilated main duct

The correct answer is (**d**). Dilated main duct in the setting of a side branch IPMN indicates a combined type IPMN and is at high risk for malignancy. Endoscopic ultrasound is indicated to work up the lesion.

2. Which of the following differentiates an IPMN from a mucinous tumor?
   a) Absence of ovarian type stroma
   b) Connection with the main pancreatic duct
   c) Presence of mucin
   d) Nodular enhancing components

The correct answer is (**a**). Side branch IPMNs are lined with columnar cells with abundant intracellular mucin. Some mucinous tumors can communicate with the pancreatic duct. Malignant side branch IPMNs can have nodular enhancing components.

■ Case 37

1. Which of the following pancreatic duct diameter is a strong predictor of malignancy?
   a) 1 to 3 mm
   b) 3 to 5 mm
   c) 5 to 10 mm
   d) ≥ 10 mm

The correct answer is (**d**). A main pancreatic duct ≥ 10 mm has 78% sensitivity for malignancy.

2. Which of the following patients requires MRCP follow-up?
   a) Main pancreatic duct diameter < 5 mm
   b) Enhancing mural nodule
   c) Thick pancreatic duct wall
   d) Duct diameter > 10 mm

The correct answer is (**a**). A pancreatic duct < 5 mm in diameter can be followed with MRCP for changes in 2 years.

■ Case 38

1. The most common functioning PNET is:
   a) Gastrinoma
   b) Insulinoma
   c) Glucanoma
   d) VIPoma

The correct answer is (**b**). Insulinomas are the most common functioning endocrine neoplasm of the pancreas. Over 90% of them are benign.

2. Which of the following genetic syndromes have the highest incidence of PNETs?
   a) Neurofibromatosis type 1
   b) Von Hippel-Lindau disease
   c) Tuberous sclerosis complex
   d) Multiple endocrine neoplasia type I

The correct answer is (**d**). Multiple endocrine neoplasia type I has the highest risk of developing a pancreatic neuroendocrine neoplasm.

■ Case 39

1. Venous drainage from an accessory spleen goes to:
   a) The splenic vein
   b) A mesenteric vein
   c) The superior mesenteric vein
   d) The portal vein

The correct answer is (**a**). An accessory spleen has venous drainage into the splenic vein like the spleen.

2. Which is the most common location for an accessory spleen?
   a) Pancreatic tail
   b) Inferior and medial to the spleen
   c) Lateral to the spleen
   d) Superior to the spleen

The correct answer is (**b**). The most common site for an accessory spleen is inferior and medial to the spleen. The second most common site is in the pancreatic tail. Almost no accessory splenic tissue is found lateral or superior to the spleen.

■ Case 40

1. Pancreas divisum is diagnosed when:
   a) The ventral duct crosses the CBD anteriorly to drain into the minor papilla
   b) The ventral duct crosses the CBD anteriorly to drain into the major papilla
   c) The dorsal duct crosses the CBD anteriorly to drain into the minor papilla
   d) The dorsal duct crosses the CBD anteriorly to drain into the major papilla

The correct answer is (**a**). Pancreas divisum occurs when the ventral duct (main pancreatic duct) crosses the CBD anteriorly and drains via the minor papilla (Santorini).

2. Which of the following modalities is best used to diagnose pancreas divisum?
   a) MRCP
   b) MRCP with secretin
   c) Pancreas CT
   d) ERCP

The correct answer is (**b**). MRCP with secretin has a sensitivity of 86% compared to MRCP alone (52%). The administration of secretin provides ductal dilation, enabling detection.

■ Case 41

1. The appropriate management of a suspected mucinous cystic neoplasm of the pancreas is:
   a) Follow-up MRI in 12 months
   b) Referral for surgical resection
   c) Endoscopic ultrasound
   d) Endoscopic retrograde cholangiopancreatography

The correct answer is (**b**). Referral for surgical resection is appropriate. Not all parts of the wall of a mucinous cystic pancreatic neoplasm may have the cellular atypia or malignant change. Therefore, biopsy is unreliable and surgical excision en bloc is the preferred method of treatment.

2. Which of the following is present in a mucinous cystic neoplasm?
   a) Mucin
   b) Nodular enhancement
   c) Ovarian stroma
   d) Septae

The correct answer is (**c**). The presence of ovarian stroma is seen in mucinous cystic tumors of the pancreas. Intraductal papillary mucinous neoplasm lack the ovarian-like stroma although they contain mucin and can have enhancing nodules and septae.

■ Case 42

1. The most common specific imaging feature of acinar cell carcinoma is that:
   a) Lesions are usually cystic
   b) Lesions are usually infiltrative
   c) Lesions are usually exophytic
   d) Lesions are usually hyperenhancing

The correct answer is (**c**). In a series and the author's experience, this rare lesion is usually exophytic compared to other pancreatic lesions.

2. The most common cell type in the pancreas is:
   a) Acinar cells
   b) Ductal epithelial cells
   c) Islet cells
   d) Alpha cells

The correct answer is (**a**). The most common cell in the pancreas is the acinar cell, comprising about 80%; nevertheless, acinar cell carcinoma is a rare tumor forming only about 1% of pancreatic neoplasms.

■ Case 43

1. Annular pancreas occurs due to:
   a) Incomplete rotation of the dorsal anlage
   b) Incomplete rotation of the ventral anlage
   c) Incomplete formation of the dorsal anlage
   d) Incomplete formation of the ventral anlage

The correct answer is (**b**). Annular pancreas is due to incomplete rotation of the ventral anlage.

2. In the extramural type, the annular duct joins the:
   a) MPD
   b) The common bile duct
   c) The duodenum
   d) The stomach

The correct answer is (**a**). In the extramural type, the annular duct joins the main pancreatic duct.

■ Case 44

1. Which of the following modalities is best suited for evaluating suspected focal fatty infiltration that appears like a pancreatic mass?
   a) Magnetic resonance imaging/magnetic resonance cholangiopancreatography of the pancreas
   b) CT of the pancreas
   c) Ultrasound of the pancreas
   d) Endoscopic retrograde cholangiopancreatography of the pancreas

The correct answer is (**a**). Magnetic resonance imaging/magnetic resonance cholangiopancreatography is the best modality to evaluate fatty masses, especially when they are small and admixed with pancreatic tissue. In-/opposed-phase imaging and T1 pre- and fat-saturated images can confidently identify fat.

2. Which of the following areas are spared from fatty infiltration in all types of regional pancreatic lipomatosis?
   a) Head of the pancreas
   b) Body of the pancreas
   c) Uncinate process of the pancreas
   d) Peribiliary region

The correct answer is (**d**). In all types, the peribiliary region is spared from fatty change. This can serve as an important landmark in evaluating patients with pancreatic lipomatosis.

■ Case 45

1. Which of the following serum markers helps in the diagnosis of AIP type 1?
   a) IgA
   b) IgG2
   c) IgE
   d) IgG4

The correct answer is (**d**). AIP type 1 is associated with increased serum IgG4 and plasma cell infiltrates in the pancreas.

2. A patient presents with pancreatitis on CT associated with biliary obstruction and an inconclusive pancreatic biopsy. Which of the following would help with the diagnosis?
   a) Perform an MRI/MRCP
   b) Repeat imaging after course of corticosteroids
   c) Perform an endoscopic retrograde cholangiopancreatography
   d) Perform an open pancreatic biopsy

The correct answer is (**b**). Both forms of AIP respond well to corticosteroids. After treatment, improvement by imaging and symptoms is useful in establishing the diagnosis. Patients with AIP type 1 tend to relapse and may need chronic corticosteroid treatment.

■ Case 46

1. Which of the following imaging findings helps in the diagnosis of SPEN?
    a) Calcifications
    b) Hemorrhage and fibrous capsule
    c) Arterial enhancement
    d) Delayed enhancement

The correct answer is (**b**). Large masses with hemorrhage, solid and cystic areas, and a fibrous capsule are imaging findings typical of a pancreatic SPEN.

2. The preferred treatment of a SPEN is:
    a) Surgical en bloc resection
    b) Radiation
    c) Chemotherapy
    d) Imaging follow-up

The correct answer is (**a**). Solid and papillary epithelial neoplasm of the pancreas is treated by surgical resection with good outcomes.

■ Case 47

1. Which of the following is a feature of a splenic pseudocyst (secondary)?
    a) Have an epithelial lining
    b) Have septations
    c) Can change in size over time
    d) Have peripheral calcifications

The correct answer is (**d**). Splenic pseudocysts, which are formed after trauma or infection, have wall calcification.

2. Which of the following therapies can be used for symptomatic nonparasitic splenic cysts?
    a) Total splenectomy
    b) Partial splenectomy
    c) Embolization
    d) Drainage

The correct answer is (**d**). Percutaneous or surgical drainage of symptomatic splenic cysts can be performed.

■ Case 48

1. Which of the following would be a contraindication to percutaneous drain placement?
    a) Size > 5 cm
    b) Well-formed capsule with a unilocular abscess
    c) Size < 3 cm
    d) Some hemorrhage in the lesion

The correct answer is (**c**). Splenic abscesses are readily drained with percutaneous drainage catheter. Smaller lesions are usually aspirated without drain placement. All other choices are favorable to drain placement.

2. Which of the following cases require surgical intervention?
    a) Splenic abscess that collapses on aspiration
    b) Splenic abscess with a drain that has decreasing output
    c) Persistent fever, elevated white blood cell count, and pain despite antibiotics and drainage
    d) Large unilocular abscess

The correct answer is (**c**). Persistent fever despite drainage and antibiotics may require surgical resection.

■ Case 49

1. Which of the following can mimic a subacute splenic hematoma?
    a) Splenic abscess
    b) Metastasis
    c) Splenomegaly
    d) Sickle cell disease

The correct answer is (**a**). Splenic abscess can have similar imaging features of an evolving hematoma. Patient history is important in the interpretation of the study.

2. Which of the following is important in management of a splenic hematoma?
    a) Prompt percutaneous drainage
    b) Splenectomy
    c) Imaging to identify acute hemorrhage and splenic rupture
    d) Correction of coagulopathy

The correct answer is (**c**). Imaging to rule out expansion of the hematoma and rupture of the spleen is important in the conservative management.

■ Case 50

1. Splenic metastases imaged at portal venous phase:
   a) Enhance greater than the splenic parenchyma
   b) Enhance about the same as splenic parenchyma
   c) Enhance less than splenic parenchyma
   d) Do not show any enhancement

The correct answer is (c). Most splenic metastases are hypoenhancing relative to splenic parenchyma on portal venous phase images.

2. Which of the following are signs of benignity of splenic lesions?
   a) Solitary lesion
   b) Multiple lesions
   c) Newly developing lesions
   d) Fluid-attenuating lesion with peripheral calcification

The correct answer is (d). Fluid-attenuating lesion with peripheral calcification would be an imaging feature of a splenic pseudocyst.

■ Case 51

1. The treatment for splenic infarctions is:
   a) Pain control and correcting the underlying cause
   b) Catheter administration of tissue plasminogen activator
   c) Splenectomy
   d) Repeat imaging

The correct answer is (a). Most symptomatic splenic infarctions require only pain control and reversal of the underlying cause. In cases such as sickle cell disease, patients are managed with pain control and monitoring for infection.

2. The outcomes for isolated splenic infractions are:
   a) Very good with most patients completely recovering
   b) Poor with patients requiring splenectomy
   c) Dependent on vaccinations administered after infarctions
   d) Variable, depending on the age of the patient

The correct answer is (a). Most patients with splenic infarctions recover well. Patients with splenic infarctions from a hematologic malignancy have worse outcomes.

■ Case 52

1. The majority of patients with a grade 3 splenic laceration need:
   a) Emergent splenic artery coil embolization
   b) Particle embolization
   c) Observation and follow-up imaging
   d) Splenectomy

The correct answer is (c). The majority of patients (about 80%) with a grade 3 laceration can be successfully managed conservatively. This decreases to about 15% in patients with a grade 5 laceration.

2. Which of the following features would require embolization?
   a) Presence of a 3 cm laceration
   b) Presence of a 5 cm laceration
   c) Subcapsular hematoma
   d) Active contrast extravasation and dropping hematocrit

The correct answer is (d). Imaging findings such as contrast extravasation or direct evidence of vascular injury such as pseudoaneurysm/arteriovenous fistula in a patient with clinical signs of ongoing bleeding are candidates for embolization.

■ Case 53

1. The threshold treatment size for a splenic artery pseudoaneurysm is:
   a) 1 cm
   b) 2 cm
   c) 3 cm
   d) 4 cm

The correct answer is (b). Splenic artery pseudoaneurysms > 2 cm have higher rates of rupture and need to be treated electively. All leaking and newly formed pseudoaneurysms are treated. Without intervention, rupture mortality can approach 90%.

2. Which of the following is a sign the pseudoaneurysm can be monitored and not treated?
   a) New pseudoaneurysm
   b) Peripheral calcification
   c) Size < 2 cm
   d) Location in the splenic artery

The correct answer is (c). Chronic pseudoaneurysm < 2 cm can be followed. Calcification of the wall and location of the pseudoaneurysm is not indicative of a higher risk of rupture.

■ Case 54

1. Siderotic splenic nodules are associated with:
   a) Carcinoma
   b) Splenic infarctions
   c) Splenic infections
   d) Portal hypertension

The correct answer is (**d**). Siderotic nodules of the spleen are associated with portal hypertension, portal or splenic vein thrombosis, hemolytic anemia, leukemia, lymphoma, repeated blood transfusions, hemochromatosis, and paroxysmal nocturnal hemoglobinuria.

2. The best imaging test for detection of siderotic nodules of the spleen is:
   a) Plain film of the abdomen
   b) CT of the abdomen
   c) In-/opposed-phase MRI of the abdomen
   d) Ultrasound of the spleen

The correct answer is (**c**). The iron contained in the nodules produces a blooming artifact that is easily detected at MRI.

■ Case 55

1. The imaging findings that are suggestive of SANT are:
   a) F18-FDG avidity
   b) Hypoenhancing splenic mass
   c) Multiple lesions
   d) Lesion is hypointense on T2 MRI with hemorrhage

The correct answer is (**d**). SANTs, unlike other splenic lesions, are characteristically T2-hypointense. The other imaging features are not helpful in differentiating them from malignant lesions.

2. The histologic findings in SANT consist of:
   a) Vascular nodules surrounded by concentric collagen fibers or fibrinoid rim
   b) Cystic spaces lined with unilayered or multilayered endothelium
   c) Fibrous septa separated by proliferating vascular channels, which are lined with flat endothelial cells
   d) Red pulp elements in a disorganized fashion, with scant fibrous trabeculae

The correct answer is (**a**). Histologically sclerosing angiomatoid nodular transformation is composed of vascular nodules surrounded by concentric collagen fibers or fibrinoid rim.

■ Case 56

1. A 40-year-old with a < 2 cm splenic hemangioma. The lesion is best:
   a) Resected
   b) Embolized
   c) Biopsied
   d) Followed

The correct answer is (**d**). Small splenic hemangiomas are safely followed as rupture is rare.

2. Splenic hemangiomas are considered:
   a) Fibrous lesions
   b) Congenital lesions
   c) Malignant lesions
   d) Cystic lesions

The correct answer is (**b**). Splenic hemangiomas are congenital, solid vascular lesions

■ Case 57

1. In heterotaxy syndrome, venous drainage from the lower extremity to the chest occurs via:
   a) Supra renal IVC
   b) Hepatic IVC
   c) Azygous vein
   d) Venous collaterals

The correct answer is (**c**). The syndrome is characterized by venous drainage via the azygous vein, which drains the infrarenal IVC.

2. The most consistent findings in heterotaxy syndrome are:
   a) Polysplenia and a preduodenal portal vein
   b) Central liver and a right gastric bubble
   c) Intestinal malrotation and polysplenia
   d) Polysplenia and IVC interruption

The correct answer is (**d**). Polysplenia and IVC interruption are the most consistent abdominal findings.

■ Case 58

1. Which of the following is the most specific sign of appendiceal rupture?
   a) Extraluminal appendicolith
   b) Ileus
   c) Pelvis abscess
   d) Appendiceal wall enhancement

The correct answer is (**a**). Extraluminal appendicolith is the most specific sign of appendiceal rupture because there is frank spillage of appendiceal contents into the abdomen.

2. The treatment in cases of appendiceal rupture and abscess formation is:
   a) Surgical appendectomy
   b) Image-guided drainage of the abscess
   c) Antibiotics alone
   d) Surgical partial colectomy

The correct answer is (**b**). In cases of appendiceal rupture, drainage of the abscess is first attempted in conjunction with antibiotics to decrease the inflammation and drain the infected collection.

■ Case 59

1. Which of the following is the accepted treatment of a mucinous appendiceal neoplasm?
   a) Appendectomy
   b) Right hemicolectomy
   c) Antibiotics
   d) Drainage

The correct answer is (**b**). Correct diagnosis of appendiceal mucinous neoplasms is important as the management differs significantly from the management of acute appendicitis. The surgical treatment is a right hemicolectomy to remove the diseased appendix without spillage and intraperitoneal spread.

2. Which of the following is the modality of choice in evaluating a mucinous appendiceal neoplasm?
   a) CT scan of the abdomen with oral and intravenous contrast
   b) MRI of the abdomen with intravenous contrast
   c) F18–fluorodeoxyglucose positron emission tomography/CT of the abdomen and pelvis
   d) Colonoscopy

The correct answer is (**a**). CT scan of the abdomen and pelvis is the standard imaging modality. F18–fluorodeoxyglucose positron emission tomography/CT is not used due to its low sensitivity caused by hypocellularity of the tumor. MRI is used, occasionally, but is not the first line imaging modality. Colonoscopy has a low sensitivity to detect appendiceal adenocarcinoma.

■ Case 60

1. Which of the modalities has the best sensitivity to detect peritoneal carcinomatosis?
   a) Contrast-enhanced CT
   b) F18-fluorodeoxyglucose PET/CT
   c) MRI with DWI
   d) ¹¹¹In-octreotide

The correct answer is (**c**). MRI of the abdomen and pelvis that includes DWI has shown the highest sensitivity to detect peritoneal disease and implants. DWI is able to differentiate between bulk water and mucinous deposits that show restricted diffusion.

2. Which of the following, if seen, is most consistently an appendiceal carcinoma?
   a) Ascites
   b) Peritoneal nodularity
   c) Infiltrative appendiceal soft tissue mass
   d) Small bowel obstruction

The correct answer is (**c**). Infiltrative soft tissue mass involving the appendix should be considered appendiceal carcinoma. Other findings include appendiceal cystic dilatation with a diameter > 15 mm.

■ Case 61

1. The most common site for a gastrointestinal neuroendocrine neoplasm is the:
   a) Small bowel
   b) Colon
   c) Esophagus
   d) Rectum

The correct answer is (**a**). The small bowel is the most common site for gastrointestinal neuroendocrine tumors, and within the small bowel, the ileum is the most common location. About 31% of neuroendocrine tumors occur in the small bowel.

2. The most common tumor of the appendix is:
   a) Lymphoma
   b) Adenocarcinoma
   c) Adenoma
   d) Neuroendocrine tumor

The correct answer is (**d**). Neuroendocrine tumors are the most common tumors of the appendix, accounting for about 50% of lesions.

■ Case 62

1. Which of the following is the most specific imaging finding for esophageal leiomyoma?
   a) Central necrosis
   b) Low-level enhancement
   c) Smooth border
   d) Calcification

The correct answer is (**d**). The presence of calcification is very specific for the entity. Esophageal leiomyoma tends to have midlevel enhancement with smooth borders.

2. Which of the following is most likely to be detected with esophageal leiomyoma?
   a) Reflux disease
   b) Achalasia
   c) Hiatal hernia
   d) Luminal obstruction

The correct answer is (**c**). Hiatal hernia is the most common additional finding in patients with esophageal leiomyoma.

■ Case 63

1. What is the upper limit on plain film radiography for gastric band slippage?
   a) 30 degrees
   b) 48 degrees
   c) 58 degrees
   d) 68 degrees

The correct answer is (**c**). Gastric band should have a Phi angle < 60 degrees, with a range from 4 to 58 degrees.

2. The most sensitive and specific sign of gastric band slippage is:
   a) Abnormal Phi angle > 58 degrees
   b) A distended pouch
   c) Inferior displacement of the band
   d) The O-Sign

The correct answer is (**c**). Inferior displacement of the su-perolateral band margin by > 2.4 cm from the diaphragm was 95% sensitive and 97–98% specific for the diagnosis.

■ Case 64

1. The most common cause of a colovesical fistula is:
   a) Colon adenocarcinoma
   b) Bladder adenocarcinoma
   c) Diverticular disease
   d) Fistulizing Crohn's disease

The correct answer is (**c**). The most common cause of colovesical fistula is diverticular disease with a reported incidence ranging from 2 to 23%.

2. The most common clinical symptom in a patient with suspected colovesical fistula is:
   a) Fecaluria
   b) Pneumaturia
   c) Pain
   d) Sepsis

The correct answer is (**b**). Pneumaturia is present in about 71% of patients with a suspected colovesical fistula. The presence of pneumaturia and fecaluria is pathognomonic.

■ Case 65

1. The most specific finding of epiploic appendagitis is:
   a) Fatty mass with hyperattenuating rim
   b) Pericolonic fatty mass
   c) Pericolonic inflammation
   d) Central dot in a pericolonic fatty mass

The correct answer is (**a**). The fatty mass with hyperatten-uating rim is the most specific finding. Inflammation and central area of high attenuation due to venous thrombosis is supportive if present.

2. The treatment for epiploic appendagitis is:
   a) Resection of the lesion
   b) Treatment of symptoms
   c) Bowel rest
   d) Antibiotic therapy

The correct answer is (**b**). Epiploic appendagitis is a self-limiting illness that can be managed conservatively with adequate pain control. The use of antibiotics or surgery is not necessary as the findings on CT tend to be pathognomonic.

■ Case 66

1. The most accurate sign at computed tomography for pseudomembranous colitis is:
   a) Ascites
   b) Nodular colonic wall thickening
   c) Severe colonic wall edema
   d) Mucosal hyperemia

The correct answer is (**c**). Colonic wall edema is an ac-curate sign for pseudomembranous colitis. Trapped oral contrast in the folds produces the accordion sign and thumbprinting on radiography.

2. The most severe complication that necessitates surgery is:
   a) Ascites
   b) Free air in the abdomen
   c) Dilated bowel loops
   d) Mucosal hyperemia

The correct answer is (**b**). Toxic megacolon and colonic perforation are severe complications that have high mortality and necessitate surgical intervention.

■ Case 67

1. The most common type of giant colonic diverticulum is:
   a) Type 1: a pseudodiverticulum
   b) Type 2: a walled-off abscess
   c) Type 3: a true diverticulum with all wall layers
   d) Unclassified type

The correct answer is (**b**). About two thirds of giant colonic diverticula lack a true wall and have a fibrous wall that likely forms from a contained perforation and abscess.

2. The most common location for giant colonic diverticulum is:
   a) The sigmoid colon
   b) The descending colon
   c) The ascending colon
   d) The cecum

The correct answer is (**a**). The most common site for a giant colonic diverticulum is the sigmoid, presumably because the sigmoid is the most frequent site of diverticulitis.

■ Case 68

1. The cause for buried bumper syndrome is:
   a) Large bore catheter
   b) Rubber balloon fixator
   c) Tight external fixator
   d) Endoscopic placement

The correct answer is (**c**). A tight external fixator and a rigid or semirigid internal fixator are the main cause for the entity. The entity can also occur with a balloon catheter. Other risk factors include malignancy, poor nutritional status, and weight gain.

2. Which of the following is an accurate sign of a buried bumper?
   a) Occlusion of the tube
   b) Immobility of the fixator device
   c) Redness around the site
   d) Pain around the site

The correct answer is (**b**). A buried bumper is fixed in the body wall and is not mobile. Occlusion of the tube lumen can occur for other reasons. Redness and pain are not specific.

■ Case 69

1. The most common volvulus of the colon is:
   a) Cecal volvulus
   b) Sigmoid volvulus
   c) Transverse colon volvulus
   d) Cecal bascule

The correct answer is (**b**). Sigmoid volvulus is the most common volvulus, accounting for about 60% of cases. About 30% are cecal volvulus, and about 2% are transverse colonic volvulus.

2. Which of the following is a sign of necrosis?
   a) Sigmoid colon distention
   b) Frothy fecal matter in the colonic segment
   c) Hyperdensity in the wall of the affected segment
   d) Mesenteric edema about the swirled vessels

The correct answer is (**c**). Hyperdensity in the wall segment indicates hemorrhagic necrosis with blood products in the wall of the colonic segment.

■ Case 70

1. Which of the following type of cecal volvulus needs surgical attention?
   a) Cecum fixed in the pelvis due to adhesions
   b) Cecum distended and displaced to the left upper abdomen with a mesenteric swirl
   c) Cecum upturned anteriorly
   d) Cecum distended and mobile across multiple exams

The correct answer is (**b**). A distended and displaced cecum with signs of volvulus needs surgery. Reports of barium enema and colonoscopy in reducing it exist, but even if successful, this treatment leaves the patient prone to repeat obstruction.

2. The presence of crossing small bowel loops around the colon indicates:
   a) Volvulus
   b) Bascule
   c) Bowel adhesions
   d) Variant anatomy

The correct answer is (**a**). The presence of crossing bowel loops anterior and posterior to the colon is a sign of cecal volvulus.

■ Case 71

1. What is purpose of oral contrast in CT colonography?
   a) Coat the colon wall
   b) Coat the polyps
   c) Tag fecal matter
   d) Outline malignant lesions

The correct answer (**c**). The use of oral contrast is to tag fecal matter. On a primary two-dimensional read, fecal matter will show dense internal contrast tagging. Care must be taken to make sure no soft tissue component is present in the polyp.

2. Which of the following lesions does not require follow-up?
   a) Tubulovillous adenoma
   b) Serrated adenoma
   c) Tubular adenoma
   d) Colonic lipoma

The correct answer is (**d**). Colonic lipoma is considered a benign lesion and does not require follow-up.

■ Case 72

1. Which of the following is correct in terms of the utilization of oral contrast?
   a) Positive oral contrast helps detect bleeding mucosal lesions
   b) Neutral oral contrast agents increase sensitivity for detecting bleeds
   c) Noncontrast CT is not needed in CTA exams for GI bleeding
   d) CTA exams for GI bleeding should be done without oral contrast

The correct answer is (**d**). CTA exams for GI bleeding should be done without oral contrast. The presence of neutral oral contrast diminishes the sensitivity of the study. The noncontrast phase helps detect any retained hyperdense material in the colon that may be mistaken for a bleed.

2. The most common cause of lower GI bleeding is:
   a) Diverticular bleed
   b) Colonic adenocarcinoma
   c) Colonic ischemia
   d) Colonic polyps

The correct answer is (**a**). The most common cause of lower GI bleeding is diverticular disease.

■ Case 73

1. Which of the following findings are concerning for secondary achalasia?
   a) An acute onset of symptoms
   b) Tram-track appearance of the contrast column in the narrowed area
   c) Smooth tapering of the affected segment
   d) Corkscrew appearance with spasm

The correct answer is (**a**). Secondary achalasia has a shorter duration of symptoms, usually a few months.

2. Which of the following is a characteristic finding in primary achalasia?
   a) Smooth tapering of the dilated esophagus to a point
   b) Submucosal mass
   c) Spastic contractions
   d) Normal lower esophageal sphincter tone

The correct answer is (**a**). Smooth tapering of the dilated esophagus to a point, "bird's beak," is a characteristic finding.

■ Case 74

1. Which of the following is not a characteristic finding of esoinophilic esophagitis?
   a) Transverse lines in the esophagus that do not persist
   b) Small caliber esophagus
   c) Midesophageal strictures
   d) Proximal esophageal rings

The correct answer is (**a**). Transverse lines in the esophagus that do not persist can be present in reflux disease.

2. Which of the following is correct?
   a) Double-contrast barium esophagram is more accurate in detecting proximal esophageal rings when compared with endoscopy
   b) Double-contrast barium esophagram is more accurate in detecting esophageal exudates when compared with endoscopy
   c) Double-contrast barium esophagram is more accurate in detecting esophageal furrows when compared with endoscopy
   d) Double-contrast barium esophagram is more accurate in detecting segmental strictures when compared with endoscopy

The correct answer is (**d**). Double-contrast barium esophagram is superior to endoscopy in detecting strictures and segmental narrowing. Mucosal patterns are better detected by endoscopy.

■ Case 75

1. Specific CT sign for bowel obstruction is:
   a) Air-fluid levels
   b) Dilated small bowel ≥ 2.5 cm with a transition point
   c) Distended colon
   d) Distended stomach

The correct answer is (**b**). The most specific CT sign is small bowel dilated ≥ 2.5 cm with a transition point.

2. Most common cause of an SBO is:
   a) Adhesions
   b) Tumors
   c) Hernia
   d) Inflammatory bowel disease

The correct answer is (**a**). The most common cause of SBO is adhesions (60–70%), which are usually the result of prior abdominal surgery, whether open or laparoscopic.

■ Case 76

1. Active extravasation into the peritoneum from a liver laceration is graded as:
   a) Grade I
   b) Grade II
   c) Grade III
   d) Grade IV

The correct answer is (**d**). Active peritoneal extravasation from a liver laceration is a grade IV laceration.

2. The presence of hemobilia should suggest the presence of a:
   a) Gallbladder injury
   b) Hepatic hematoma
   c) Grade II laceration
   d) Pseudoaneurysm

The correct answer is (**d**). Pseudoaneurysm occurs in about 1% of cases. The pseudoaneurysm can decompress into the biliary tree with resultant gastrointestinal bleeding.

■ Case 77

1. Zenker's diverticulum is a:
   a) True diverticulum
   b) Traction diverticulum
   c) Pseudodiverticulum
   d) Intramural diverticulum

The correct answer is (**c**). Zenker's diverticulum is a pseudodiverticulum with herniation of the posterior pharyngeal mucosa.

2. Zenker's diverticulum herniates:
   a) Between the superior and middle pharyngeal constrictors
   b) Between the middle and inferior pharyngeal constrictors
   c) Inferior to the cricopharyngeus
   d) Between the inferior pharyngeal constrictors and the cricopharyngeus

The correct answer is (**d**). Zenker's diverticulum is a pseudodiverticulum with posterior inferior herniation of the pharyngeal mucosa between the inferior pharyngeal constrictors (thyropharyngeus) and the cricopharyngeus (the Killian triangle or Killian dehiscence). The Killian-Jamieson diverticulum herniates anteriorly inferior to the cricopharyngeus via the Killian-Jamieson space.

■ Case 78

1. Which of the following signs on a double-contrast barium esophagram suggests the stricture is malignant?
   a) Symmetric narrowing
   b) Failure to pass a barium tablet
   c) Smooth contours
   d) Irregular mucosa

The correct answer is (**d**). Irregular mucosa and asymmetric narrowing are hallmark features of a malignant esophageal stricture.

2. Which of the following is a limitation of a double-contrast barium esophagram in the follow-up imaging of a patient undergoing treatment for esophageal carcinoma?
   a) Measurement of the intraluminal mucosal mass
   b) Evaluation of the narrowed lumen of the esophagus
   c) Evaluation of the mural disease
   d) Evaluation of perforation

The correct answer is (**c**). Evaluation of mural disease, or residual mural disease, and adenopathy are poorly evaluated by esophagram and are best evaluated with endoscopy and CT.

■ Case 79

1. Which of the following findings are indicative of an organoaxial gastric volvulus?
   a) Rotation of the antrum anterosuperiorly and the fundus posteroinferiorly
   b) Rotation of the antrum posterosuperiorly and the fundus anteroinferiorly
   c) Rotation of the stomach with antrum above the gastroesophageal junction
   d) Rotation of the stomach with dilation of the fundus and collapse of the antrum

The correct answer is (**a**). In organoaxial gastric volvulus, the antrum rotates anterosuperiorly and the fundus posteroinferiorly along the long axis of the stomach.

2. Which of the following are associated with organoaxial gastric volvulus?
   a) Prior surgery
   b) Gastric bypass
   c) Billroth II procedure
   d) Diaphragmatic gastric hernia

The correct answer is (**d**). Diaphragmatic gastric hernia or eventration of the diaphragm is associated with organo-axial gastric volvulus.

■ Case 80

1. The origin of gastric GISTs is:
   a) Epithelial
   b) Mesenchymal
   c) Neural
   d) Ectodermal

The correct answer is (**b**). Gastric GISTs are mesenchymal tumors. Gastric leiomyomas also are mesenchymal tumors but lack the c-KIT mutation.

2. Large GIST tumors tend to metastasize to the:
   a) Liver
   b) Pancreas
   c) Kidney
   d) Spleen

The correct answer is (**a**). The liver and peritoneum are frequent sites of metastasis for GIST.

■ Case 81

1. The organ that is directly involved with malignancy at the gastric cardia is:
   a) The esophagus
   b) Perigastric nodes
   c) Liver
   d) Pancreas

The correct answer is (**a**). In about 60% of cases of carcinoma of the gastric cardia, the distal esophagus is involved.

2. A mucosal and submucosal tumor in the antrum and pylorus would be considered a:
   a) Polypoid: Borrmann type I
   b) Fungating: Borrmann type II
   c) Ulcerated: Borrmann type III
   d) Infiltrative: Borrmann type IV

The correct answer is (**d**). The distal stomach infiltrative tumor is characterized as a Borrmann type IV lesion. It can have features of linitis plastica (scirrhous tumor).

■ Case 82

1. Which of the following indicates the gastric ulcer is malignant?
   a) Smooth ulcer crater
   b) Irregular ulcer crater
   c) Gastric folds radiating toward the ulcer
   d) Ulcer that projects deep to the gastric mucosa

The correct answer is (**b**). Malignant ulcers have an irregular ulcer crater and are eccentric to the soft tissue mound around the ulcer.

2. Which of the following is a sign the ulcer is malignant?
   a) Soft tissue around the ulcer that is convex toward the stomach
   b) Deep ulcer base
   c) Smooth thickening around the ulcer edge
   d) Collection of barium that is persistent

The correct answer is (**a**). Soft tissue surrounding the ulcer that is irregular and convex towards the stomach lumen is a finding suspicious for malignancy.

■ Case 83

1. Which of the following is considered an abnormal aortomesenteric angle?
   a) Angle 15 to 22 degrees
   b) Angle 25 to 30 degrees
   c) Angle 30 to 45 degrees
   d) Angle > 45 degrees

The correct answer is (**a**). An abnormal aortomesenteric angle is considered an angle < 22 to 25 degrees.

2. Which of the following is an upper gastrointestinal barium finding in SMA syndrome?
   a) A high ligament of Treitz
   b) A patulous duodenum
   c) Distended stomach
   d) Obstruction of the duodenum at L3 with antiperistaltic flow

The correct answer is (**d**). Failure of passage of contrast across the transverse portion of the duodenum and antiperistaltic flow are findings in SMA syndrome.

■ Case 84

1. Which of the following types of polyp is predominant in PJS?
   a) Fundic gland polyps
   b) Hyperplastic polyps
   c) Adenomatous polyps
   d) Hamartomatous polyps

The correct answer is (**d**). PJS is characterized by hamartomatous polyps (Peutz–Jeghers type) of the gastrointestinal tract and melanocytic mucocutaneous hyperpigmentation.

2. Which of the following locations is most common for polyps in PJS?
   a) Small bowel
   b) Colon
   c) Stomach
   d) Esophagus

The correct answer is (**a**). The small bowel is the most frequent site of polyps; small bowel polyps occur in about 64% of patients with PJS.

■ Case 85

1. Which of the following is a predictor that the mass is an ampullary tumor?
   a) Tapering of the distal CBD
   b) Nodular mass at the major papilla
   c) Nodular mass in the distal CBD
   d) Bulging of the pancreatic head

The correct answer is (**b**). A nodular mass at the major papilla suggests an ampullary tumor. Tapering of the distal CBD suggests a benign stricture. A nodular mass in the distal CBD is most suggestive of a distal CBD cholangiocarcinoma. Bulging of the pancreatic head indicates a pancreatic mass such as an adenocarcinoma.

2. Which of the following is the reason ampullary masses are detected earlier?
   a) Duodenal obstruction is common
   b) Pancreatitis is common
   c) Biliary obstruction is common leading to work-up
   d) Patients present with malabsorption syndrome

The correct answer is (**c**). Ampullary carcinomas present earlier than periampullary masses as about 75% produce biliary obstruction and early jaundice.

■ Case 86

1. Which of the following are early signs of impending perforation in SC?
   a) Rectal distention
   b) Fecaloma
   c) Rectal wall thickening
   d) Discontinuous mucosa

The correct answer is (**d**). Although all the findings are present in SC, the discontinuous mucosa indicates early perforation due to pressure erosion of the colon caused by the fecaloma.

2. The reason for colonic perforation in SC is:
   a) Increased colonic wall pressure from the fecaloma
   b) Thickened rectal wall causing ischemia
   c) Distention of the rectum leading to decreased vascular perfusion
   d) Localized infection caused by stool retention

The correct answer is (**a**). The most significant risk in SC is colonic perforation due to pressure erosion of the wall that results in ulceration and ultimately perforation caused by the fecaloma.

■ Case 87

1. Which of the following is more commonly associated with lymphoma of the bowel than adenocarcinoma?
    a) Nodal disease and splenomegaly
    b) Infiltrative soft tissue in the mesentery
    c) Bowel obstruction
    d) EBV negative status

The correct answer is (**a**). Although primary small bowel lymphoma can present as a discrete mass and no nodal disease, the presence of bulky nodal disease and spleno- megaly is more suggestive of lymphoma.

2. EBV-related Burkitt's lymphoma most commonly occurs at which site in the pediatric population?
    a) Duodenum
    b) Jejunum
    c) Ileum
    d) Ileocecal valve

The correct answer is (**d**). The ileocecal valve is the most common site of disease in pediatric EBV-related Burkitt's lymphoma.

■ Case 88

1. For ACE inhibitor-induced angioedema, the most common site of involvement is the:
    a) Duodenum
    b) Jejunum
    c) Ileum
    d) Colon

The correct answer is (**b**). The jejunum alone is involved in about 50% of the cases of ACE inhibitor–induced angioedema. The ileum alone is next most common and a jejunal plus ileal pattern is the least common.

2. Which of the following is a mimic of ACE inhibitor- induced angioedema?
    a) Mesenteric venous ischemia
    b) Peptic ulcer disease
    c) Chronic radiation enteritis
    d) Lymphoma

The correct answer is (**a**). Acute mesenteric venous isch- emia mimics ACE inhibitor–induced angioedema with sub- mucosal wall edema and hyperenhancement of the serosa and mucosa due to preserved arterial function.

■ Case 89

1. Which of the following tests is the best in patients suspected of PI?
    a) Plain film radiography
    b) Barium examination
    c) Ultrasound
    d) CT

The correct answer is (**d**). CT is the best modality to evalu- ate PI. It far exceeds the accuracy of plain films, ultrasound, and MRI in the acutely ill patient.

2. Which of the following findings indicate an acute, life- threatening condition in a patient with PI?
    a) Gas throughout the colon wall
    b) Dependent ascites
    c) Thrombus in superior mesenteric artery
    d) Immunocompromised patient

The correct answer is (**c**). Thrombus in the superior mes- enteric artery and PI indicates ischemia and can be acutely life-threatening.

■ Case 90

1. The most significant complication from a closed-loop obstruction is:
    a) Lactic acidosis
    b) Bowel ischemia and perforation
    c) Vomiting and aspiration
    d) Organ failure

The correct answer is (**b**). The major complication from a closed loop obstruction is strangulation further compli- cated by bowel ischemia, which has high mortality.

2. Which of the following is a specific sign of closed-loop obstruction?
    a) Dilated loops of bowel
    b) Attenuated mesenteric vessels
    c) Interloop fluid
    d) Dilated small bowel loop in a C- or U-shaped configuration

The correct answer is (**d**). The configuration of small bowel loops in a C or U shape is a specific sign as the afferent and efferent sites of obstruction are visualized. The other findings can be present in simple bowel obstructions and bowel ischemia.

■ Case 91

1. Which of the following would be classified as a hepatopetal shunt?
   a) Shunt from the splenic vein to the left renal vein
   b) Shunt from the portal system to the pelvic veins
   c) Shunt from the left gastric vein to the esophageal venous plexus
   d) Venous collaterals in the periportal region

The correct answer is (**d**). Collaterals in the periportal region alongside the thrombosed portal vein form pathways to the liver parenchyma.

2. The leading cause of portal venous thrombosis is:
   a) Cirrhosis
   b) Polycythemia
   c) Appendicitis
   d) Abdominal surgery

The correct answer is (**a**). It is estimated up to 15% of adults with cirrhosis awaiting transplantation have portal venous thrombosis.

■ Case 92

1. Which of the following is true of a nonleadpoint intussusception?
   a) They are transient
   b) Bowel obstruction is commonly present
   c) Treatment is necessary
   d) They are common

The correct answer is (**a**). Nonleadpoint intussusceptions are rare and are transient without bowel wall edema or obstruction and do not require treatment.

2. Which of the following is the most common colocolic leadpoint mass for intussusception in adults?
   a) Adenocarcinoma
   b) Venous malformations
   c) Lipoma
   d) Lymphoma

The correct answer is (**c**). Lipomas are the most common benign cause of colocolic intussusception in adults.

■ Case 93

1. The most common location for primary omental torsion is the:
   a) Right lower quadrant
   b) Left lower quadrant
   c) Perihepatic omentum
   d) Perisplenic omentum

The correct answer is (**a**). The most common area of primary omental torsion is the right lower quadrant where the omentum is redundant.

2. The treatment for omental infarction is:
   a) Surgery
   b) Biopsy
   c) Pain control
   d) Repeat imaging

The correct answer is (**c**). After confident diagnosis has been made, the treatment for omental infarction is pain control. Most cases resolve as the area of fat necrosis decreases in size.

■ Case 94

1. Which of the following is considered specific finding in celiac disease?
   a) Mesenteric nodes
   b) Bowel wall thickening
   c) Reversal of jejunal and ileal fold pattern
   d) Small bowel intussusception

The correct answer is (**c**). The reversal of the jejunal and ileal fold pattern is a specific finding. The ileum assumes a jejunal fold pattern and the jejunum, due to villous atrophy, has a bland appearance. The other findings can be found in other entities.

2. The cause of celiac disease is:
   a) Autoimmune disease from ingestion of gluten proteins
   b) Idiopathic inflammatory condition of the small bowel
   c) *Mycobacterium avium* infection
   d) Malignancy-related bowel complex

The correct answer is (**a**). Celiac disease is a chronic immune-mediated inflammatory enteropathy caused by gluten exposure in genetically susceptible individuals. It affects about 1 in 200 persons in the United States.

■ Case 95

1. Which of the following is the most common finding in VHL syndrome?
    a) Pancreatic cysts
    b) Renal cell carcinoma
    c) Pancreatic neuroendocrine tumors
    d) Pheochromocytoma

The correct answer is (**a**). Pancreatic cysts are the most common finding in VHL syndrome with about 50 to 91% of patients having the finding.

2. Which of the following lesions associated with VHL syndrome requires annual screening?
    a) Serous cystadenoma of the pancreas
    b) Renal cysts
    c) Renal cell carcinoma
    d) Pancreatic neuroendocrine neoplasm

The correct answer is (**c**). Although the renal cell carcinomas of VHL syndrome are slow growing, they can metastasize and are treated with ablation or surgery.

■ Case 96

1. Which of following is a characteristic pattern of enhancement in carcinoid tumors?
    a) Poor arterial enhancement
    b) Portal venous enhancement
    c) Arterial hyperenhancement
    d) Early washout

The correct answer is (**c**). Typical carcinoid tumors show avid arterial enhancement. They tend to retain contrast on delayed phases of imaging.

2. Which of the following is typical for a suspected mesenteric carcinoid?
    a) Calcification
    b) Arterial occlusion
    c) Large small bowel mass
    d) Intestinal obstruction

The correct answer is (**a**). Tumoral calcification is the most characteristic finding and can be seen in up to 70% of cases.

■ Case 97

1. Which of the following features suggest a malignant process in a mesenteric mass?
    a) Uniform enhancement
    b) Smooth border
    c) Tethering adjacent bowel
    d) Areas of tumoral necrosis

The correct answer is (**d**). Most abdominal desmoid tumors do not have necrosis. They are by nature infiltrative and can tether bowel loops.

2. The treatment of abdominal desmoid is:
    a) Chemotherapy
    b) Surgical excision
    c) Radiation
    d) Watchful waiting

The correct answer is (**b**). Tumors that are symptomatic are excised. In the setting of FAP, > 80% of patients have had prior surgery (colectomy), and prior abdominal surgery is a risk factor for developing desmoid tumors.

■ Case 98

1. The radiograph of the abdomen for exclusion of a radiopaque foreign body after surgery:
    a) Must have multiple views of the surgical site
    b) Must include the entire abdomen and pelvis
    c) Must be obtained as a spot magnified view of the surgical site
    d) Is not indicated

The correct answer is (**b**). Radiograph for radiopaque foreign body must include the entire abdomen and pelvis as there can be movement of the sponge during or after surgery.

2. The management for a gossypiboma is:
    a) Surgical removal
    b) Percutaneous drainage
    c) Follow-up if the patient is asymptomatic
    d) Notification of risk management

The correct answer is (**a**). Surgical removal is the treatment of choice for a gossypiboma as they can perforate or cause fistulae. The entity is underreported due to the potential of a medical malpractice suit. Disclosure to the patient with the help of risk management is essential.

■ Case 99

1. The most severe form of neutropenic enterocolitis can result in:
   a) Colonic wall thickening
   b) Gastrointestinal perforation
   c) Small bowel wall thickening
   d) Mesenteric inflammation

The correct answer is (**b**). Gastrointestinal perforation is the dreaded complication of neutropenic enterocolitis. Pneumatosis intestinalis, free air, and poor or nonenhancing mucosa are indicators of disease severity.

2. The most common site of involvement is:
   a) Small bowel
   b) Rectum
   c) Ascending colon
   d) Stomach

The correct answer is (**c**). The ascending colon is the most common site of involvement, often with associated involvement of the terminal ileum.

■ Case 100

1. A 35-year-old male presents with abdominal pain, weight loss, and bloody stool. If colonoscopy fails to find any pathology, the next imaging study would be:
   a) CT enterography
   b) Barium small bowel follow-through
   c) Ultrasound of the abdomen
   d) MR enterography

The correct answer is (**d**). MR enterography is an excellent modality to detect, monitor, and stage bowel inflammation. Its lack of radiation and exquisite soft tissue contrast make it good modality for monitoring the disease in young patients.

2. Which of the following is an indication of acute Crohn's disease?
   a) Bowel wall edema and mucosal hyperemia
   b) Strictures
   c) Enteroenteric fistula
   d) Fibrofatty proliferation

The correct answer is (**a**). Active disease is characterized by bowel wall edema and mucosal hyperemia. On MR imaging, active disease also restricts diffusion.

Further Readings

- ## Case 1

McEvoy SH, McCarthy CJ, Lavelle LP, et al. Hepatocellular carcinoma: illustrated guide to systematic radiologic diagnosis and staging according to guidelines of the American Association for the Study of Liver Diseases. Radiographics 2013;33(6):1653–1668

Shriki JE, Seyal AR, Dighe MK, et al. CT of Atypical and uncommon presentations of hepatocellular carcinoma. AJR Am J Roentgenol 2015;205(4):W411-23

- ## Case 2

Jha P, Poder L, Wang ZJ, Westphalen AC, Yeh BM, Coakley FV. Radiologic mimics of cirrhosis. AJR Am J Roentgenol 2010;194(4):993–999

Lee SL, Chang ED, Na SJ, et al. Pseudocirrhosis of breast cancer metastases to the liver treated by chemotherapy. Cancer Res Treat 2014;46(1):98–103

- ## Case 3

Barosa R, Pinto J, Caldeira A, Pereira E. Modern role of clinical ultrasound in liver abscess and echinococcosis. J Med Ultrason (2001) 2017;44(3):239–245

Mortelé KJ, Segatto E, Ros PR. The infected liver: radiologic-pathologic correlation. Radiographics 2004;24(4):937–955

- ## Case 4

Chung YE, Kim MJ, Park YN, et al. Varying appearances of cholangiocarcinoma: radiologic-pathologic correlation. Radiographics 2009;29(3):683–700

- ## Case 5

Dioguardi Burgio M, Ronot M, Salvaggio G, Vilgrain V, Brancatelli G. Imaging of hepatic focal nodular hyperplasia: pictorial review and diagnostic strategy. Semin Ultrasound CT MR 2016;37(6):511–524 10.1053/j.sult.2016.08.001

- ## Case 6

Tom WW, Yeh BM, Cheng JC, Qayyum A, Joe B, Coakley FV. Hepatic pseudotumor due to nodular fatty sparing: the diagnostic role of opposed-phase MRI. AJR Am J Roentgenol 2004;183(3):721–724

Venkatesh SK, Hennedige T, Johnson GB, Hough DM, Fletcher JG. Imaging patterns and focal lesions in fatty liver: a pictorial review. Abdom Radiol (NY) 2017;42(5):1374–1392

- ## Case 7

Furlan A, Marin D, Bae KT, et al. Focal liver lesions hyperintense on T1-weighted magnetic resonance images. Semin Ultrasound CT MR 2009;30(5):436–449

- ## Case 8

Kamaya A, Weinstein S, Desser TS. Multiple lesions of the spleen: differential diagnosis of cystic and solid lesions. Semin Ultrasound CT MR 2006;27(5):389–403

Mortelé KJ, Segatto E, Ros PR. The infected liver: radiologic-pathologic correlation. Radiographics 2004;24(4):937–955

- ## Case 9

Kumar N, Adam SZ, Goodhartz LA, Hoff FL, Lo AA, Miller FH. Beyond hepatic hemangiomas: the diverse appearances of gastrointestinal and genitourinary hemangiomas. Abdom Imaging 2015;40(8):3313–3329

- ## Case 10

Jang JK, Jang HJ, Kim JS, Kim TK. Focal fat deposition in the liver: diagnostic challenges on imaging. Abdom Radiol (NY) 2017;42(6):1667–1678

- ## Case 11

Venkatesh SK, Hennedige T, Johnson GB, Hough DM, Fletcher JG. Imaging patterns and focal lesions in fatty liver: a pictorial review. Abdom Radiol (NY) 2017;42(5):1374–1392

■ Case 12

Pech L, Favelier S, Falcoz MT, Loffroy R, Krause D, Cercueil JP. Imaging of Von Meyenburg complexes. Diagn Interv Imaging 2016;97(4):401–409

■ Case 13

Yang B, Chen WH, Li QY, Xiang JJ, Xu RJ. Hepatic angiomyolipoma: dynamic computed tomography features and clinical correlation. World J Gastroenterol 2009;15(27):3417–3420

■ Case 14

Tomasian A, Sandrasegaran K, Elsayes KM, Shanbhogue A, Shaaban A, Menias CO. Hematologic malignancies of the liver: spectrum of disease. Radiographics 2015;35(1):71–86

■ Case 15

Brancatelli G, Vilgrain V, Federle MP, et al. Budd-Chiari syndrome: spectrum of imaging findings. AJR Am J Roentgenol 2007;188(2):W168-76

■ Case 16

Chen MY, Bechtold RE, Savage PD. Cystic changes in hepatic metastases from gastrointestinal stromal tumors (GISTs) treated with Gleevec (imatinib mesylate). AJR Am J Roentgenol 2002;179(4):1059–1062

Sandrasegaran K, Rajesh A, Rushing DA, Rydberg J, Akisik FM, Henley JD. Gastrointestinal stromal tumors: CT and MRI findings. Eur Radiol 2005;15(7):1407–1414

■ Case 17

Grazioli L, Ambrosini R, Frittoli B, Grazioli M, Morone M. Primary benign liver lesions. Eur J Radiol 2017;95: 378–398

Wang W, Liu JY, Yang Z, et al. Hepatocellular adenoma: comparison between real-time contrast-enhanced ultrasound and dynamic computed tomography. Springerplus 2016;5(1):951

■ Case 18

Borhani AA, Wiant A, Heller MT. Cystic hepatic lesions: a review and an algorithmic approach. AJR Am J Roentgenol 2014;203(6):1192–1204

Martin DR, Kalb B, Sarmiento JM, Heffron TG, Coban I, Adsay NV. Giant and complicated variants of cystic bile duct hamartomas of the liver: MRI findings and pathological correlations. J Magn Reson Imaging 2010;31(4):903–911

■ Case 19

Costello JR, Kalb B, Chundru S, Arif H, Petkovska I, Martin DR. MR imaging of benign and malignant biliary conditions. Magn Reson Imaging Clin N Am 2014;22(3): 467–488

■ Case 20

Furlan A, Ferris JV, Hosseinzadeh K, Borhani AA. Gallbladder carcinoma update: multimodality imaging evaluation, staging, and treatment options. AJR Am J Roentgenol 2008;191(5):1440–1447

Hundal R, Shaffer EA. Gallbladder cancer: epidemiology and outcome. Clin Epidemiol 2014;6:99–109 10.2147/CLEP.S37357

■ Case 21

Bennett GL, Rusinek H, Lisi V, et al. CT findings in acute gangrenous cholecystitis. AJR Am J Roentgenol 2002;178(2):275–281

Chang WC, Sun Y, Wu EH, et al. CT findings for detecting the presence of gangrenous ischemia in cholecystitis. AJR Am J Roentgenol 2016;207(2):302–309

Corr P. Sonography of gangrenous cholecystitis. J Emerg Trauma Shock 2012;5(1):82–83

■ Case 22

Bonatti M, Vezzali N, Lombardo F, et al. Gallbladder adenomyomatosis: imaging findings, tricks and pitfalls. Insights Imaging 2017;8(2):243–253

Hammad AY, Miura JT, Turaga KK, Johnston FM, Hohenwalter MD, Gamblin TC. A literature review of radiological findings to guide the diagnosis of gallbladder adenomyomatosis. HPB (Oxford) 2016;18(2):129–135

■ Case 23

Konstantakis C, Triantos C, Theopistos V, et al. Recurrence of choledocholithiasis following endoscopic bile duct clearance: Long term results and factors associated with recurrent bile duct stones. World J Gastrointest Endosc 2017;9(1):26–33

Miller FH, Hwang CM, Gabriel H, Goodhartz LA, Omar AJ, Parsons WG III. Contrast-enhanced helical CT of choledocholithiasis. AJR Am J Roentgenol 2003;181(1):125–130

■ Case 24

Kumar A, Senthil G, Prakash A, et al. Mirizzi's syndrome: lessons learnt from 169 patients at a single center. Korean J Hepatobiliary Pancreat Surg 2016;20(1):17–22

Menias CO, Surabhi VR, Prasad SR, Wang HL, Narra VR, Chintapalli KN. Mimics of cholangiocarcinoma: spectrum of disease. Radiographics 2008;28(4):1115–1129

■ Case 25

Copelan A, Bahoura L, Tardy F, Kirsch M, Sokhandon F, Kapoor B. Etiology, diagnosis, and management of bilomas: a current update. Tech Vasc Interv Radiol 2015;18(4):236–243

Nikpour AM, Knebel RJ, Cheng D. Diagnosis and management of postoperative biliary leaks. Semin Intervent Radiol 2016;33(4):307–312

■ Case 26

Lee HK, Park SJ, Yi BH, Lee AL, Moon JH, Chang YW. Imaging features of adult choledochal cysts: a pictorial review. Korean J Radiol 2009;10(1):71–80

■ Case 27

Nayak L, Menias CO, Gayer G. Dropped gallstones: spectrum of imaging findings, complications and diagnostic pitfalls. Br J Radiol 2013;86(1028):20120588

Ramamurthy NK, Rudralingam V, Martin DF, Galloway SW, Sukumar SA. Out of sight but kept in mind: complications and imitations of dropped gallstones. AJR Am J Roentgenol 2013;200(6):1244–1253

■ Case 28

Feng X, Zheng S, Xia F, et al. Classification and management of hepatolithiasis: A high-volume, single-center's experience. Intractable Rare Dis Res 2012;1(4):151–156

Kim HJ, Kim JS, Joo MK, et al. Hepatolithiasis and intrahepatic cholangiocarcinoma: A review. World J Gastroenterol 2015;21(48):13418–13431

■ Case 29

Catalano OA, Sahani DV, Forcione DG, et al. Biliary infections: spectrum of imaging findings and management. Radiographics 2009;29(7):2059–2080

■ Case 30

Miller FH, Keppke AL, Dalal K, Ly JN, Kamler VA, Sica GT. MRI of pancreatitis and its complications: part 1, acute pancreatitis. AJR Am J Roentgenol 2004;183(6):1637–1644

Türkvatan A, Erden A, Türkoğlu MA, Seçil M, Yener Ö. Imaging of acute pancreatitis and its complications. Part 1: acute pancreatitis. Diagn Interv Imaging 2015;96(2):151–160

Türkvatan A, Erden A, Türkoğlu MA, Seçil M, Yüce G. Imaging of acute pancreatitis and its complications. Part 2: complications of acute pancreatitis. Diagn Interv Imaging 2015;96(2):161–169

■ Case 31

Duggan SN, Ní Chonchubhair HM, Lawal O, O'Connor DB, Conlon KC. Chronic pancreatitis: A diagnostic dilemma. World J Gastroenterol 2016;22(7):2304–2313

Javadi S, Menias CO, Korivi BR, et al. Pancreatic calcifications and calcified pancreatic masses: pattern recognition approach on CT. AJR Am J Roentgenol 2017;209(1):77–87

■ Case 32

Thoeni RF. The revised Atlanta classification of acute pancreatitis: its importance for the radiologist and its effect on treatment. Radiology 2012;262(3):751–764

■ Case 33

Bennett S, Lorenz JM. The role of imaging-guided percutaneous procedures in the multidisciplinary approach to treatment of pancreatic fluid collections. Semin Intervent Radiol 2012;29(4):314–318

Kim HC, Yang DM, Kim HJ, Lee DH, Ko YT, Lim JW. Computed tomography appearances of various complications associated with pancreatic pseudocysts. Acta Radiol 2008;49(7):727–734

Sheu Y, Furlan A, Almusa O, Papachristou G, Bae KT. The revised Atlanta classification for acute pancreatitis: a CT imaging guide for radiologists. Emerg Radiol 2012;19(3):237–243

■ Case 34

Dewhurst CE, Mortele KJ. Cystic tumors of the pancreas: imaging and management. Radiol Clin North Am 2012;50(3):467–486

■ Case 35

Brennan DD, Zamboni GA, Raptopoulos VD, Kruskal JB. Comprehensive preoperative assessment of pancreatic adenocarcinoma with 64-section volumetric CT. Radiographics 2007;27(6):1653–1666

Tamm EP, Balachandran A, Bhosale PR, et al. Imaging of pancreatic adenocarcinoma: update on staging/resectability. Radiol Clin North Am 2012;50(3):407–428

■ Case 36

Dewhurst CE, Mortele KJ. Cystic tumors of the pancreas: imaging and management. Radiol Clin North Am 2012;50(3):467–486

Kawamoto S, Horton KM, Lawler LP, Hruban RH, Fishman EK. Intraductal papillary mucinous neoplasm of the pancreas: can benign lesions be differentiated from malignant lesions with multidetector CT? Radiographics 2005;25(6):1451–1468, discussion 1468–1470

Yamada Y, Mori H, Matsumoto S. Intraductal papillary mucinous neoplasms of the pancreas: correlation of helical CT and dynamic MR imaging features with pathologic findings. Abdom Imaging 2008;33(4):474–481

■ Case 37

Kang HJ, Lee JM, Joo I, et al. Assessment of malignant potential in intraductal papillary mucinous neoplasms of the pancreas: comparison between multidetector CT and MR imaging with MR cholangiopancreatography. Radiology 2016;279(1):128–139

Kawamoto S, Horton KM, Lawler LP, Hruban RH, Fishman EK. Intraductal papillary mucinous neoplasm of the pancreas: can benign lesions be differentiated from malignant lesions with multidetector CT? Radiographics 2005;25(6):1451–1468, discussion 1468–1470

■ Case 38

Dromain C, Déandréis D, Scoazec JY, et al. Imaging of neuroendocrine tumors of the pancreas. Diagn Interv Imaging 2016;97(12):1241–1257

Hayashi D, Tkacz JN, Hammond S, et al. Gastroenteropancreatic neuroendocrine tumors: multimodality imaging features with pathological correlation. Jpn J Radiol 2011;29(2):85–91

Kawamoto S, Shi C, Hruban RH, et al. Small serotonin-producing neuroendocrine tumor of the pancreas associated with pancreatic duct obstruction. AJR Am J Roentgenol 2011;197(3):W482-8

■ Case 39

Kawamoto S, Johnson PT, Hall H, Cameron JL, Hruban RH, Fishman EK. Intrapancreatic accessory spleen: CT appearance and differential diagnosis. Abdom Imaging 2012;37(5):812–827

Mortelé KJ, Mortelé B, Silverman SG. CT features of the accessory spleen. AJR Am J Roentgenol 2004;183(6):1653–1657

■ Case 40

Kushnir VM, Wani SB, Fowler K, et al. Sensitivity of endoscopic ultrasound, multidetector computed tomography, and magnetic resonance cholangiopancreatography in the diagnosis of pancreas divisum: a tertiary center experience. Pancreas 2013;42(3):436–441

Rustagi T, Njei B. Magnetic resonance cholangiopancreatography in the diagnosis of pancreas divisum: a systematic review and meta-analysis. Pancreas 2014;43(6):823–828

Türkvatan A, Erden A, Türkoğlu MA, Yener Ö. Congenital variants and anomalies of the pancreas and pancreatic duct: imaging by magnetic resonance cholangiopancreaticography and multidetector computed tomography. Korean J Radiol 2013;14(6):905–913

■ Case 41

Dewhurst CE, Mortele KJ. Cystic tumors of the pancreas: imaging and management. Radiol Clin North Am 2012;50(3):467–486

Kalb B, Sarmiento JM, Kooby DA, Adsay NV, Martin DR. MR imaging of cystic lesions of the pancreas. Radiographics 2009;29(6):1749–1765

■ Case 42

Raman SP, Hruban RH, Cameron JL, Wolfgang CL, Kawamoto S, Fishman EK. Acinar cell carcinoma of the pancreas: computed tomography features—a study of 15 patients. Abdom Imaging 2013;38(1):137–143

Tatli S, Mortele KJ, Levy AD, et al. CT and MRI features of pure acinar cell carcinoma of the pancreas in adults. AJR Am J Roentgenol 2005;184(2):511–519

■ Case 43

Mortelé KJ, Rocha TC, Streeter JL, Taylor AJ. Multimodality imaging of pancreatic and biliary congenital anomalies. Radiographics 2006;26(3):715–731

Türkvatan A, Erden A, Türkoğlu MA, Yener Ö. Congenital variants and anomalies of the pancreas and pancreatic duct: imaging by magnetic resonance cholangiopancreaticography and multidetector computed tomography. Korean J Radiol 2013;14(6):905–913

■ Case 44

Mortelé KJ, Rocha TC, Streeter JL, Taylor AJ. Multimodality imaging of pancreatic and biliary congenital anomalies. Radiographics 2006;26(3):715–731

■ Case 45

Tang CSW, Sivarasan N, Griffin N. Abdominal manifestations of IgG4-related disease: a pictorial review. Insights Imaging 2018;9(4):437–448

■ Case 46

Chung EM, Travis MD, Conran RM. Pancreatic tumors in children: radiologic-pathologic correlation. Radiographics 2006;26(4):1211–1238

Rastogi A, Assing M, Taggart M, et al. Does computed tomography have the ability to differentiate aggressive from nonaggressive solid pseudopapillary neoplasm? J Comput Assist Tomogr 2018;42(3):405–411

Verde F, Fishman EK. Calcified pancreatic and peripancreatic neoplasms: spectrum of pathologies. Abdom Radiol (NY) 2017;42(11):2686–2697

■ Case 47

Karfis EA, Roustanis E, Tsimoyiannis EC. Surgical management of nonparasitic splenic cysts. JSLS 2009;13(2):207–212

Warshauer DM, Hall HL. Solitary splenic lesions. Semin Ultrasound CT MR 2006;27(5):370–388

■ Case 48

Kamaya A, Weinstein S, Desser TS. Multiple lesions of the spleen: differential diagnosis of cystic and solid lesions. Semin Ultrasound CT MR 2006;27(5):389–403

Warshauer DM, Hall HL. Solitary splenic lesions. Semin Ultrasound CT MR 2006;27(5):370–388

■ Case 49

Tonolini M, Bianco R. Nontraumatic splenic emergencies: cross-sectional imaging findings and triage. Emerg Radiol 2013;20(4):323–332

Unal E, Onur MR, Akpinar E, et al. Imaging findings of splenic emergencies: a pictorial review. Insights Imaging 2016;7(2):215–222

■ Case 50

Kamaya A, Weinstein S, Desser TS. Multiple lesions of the spleen: differential diagnosis of cystic and solid lesions. Semin Ultrasound CT MR 2006;27(5):389–403

Warshauer DM, Hall HL. Solitary splenic lesions. Semin Ultrasound CT MR 2006;27(5):370–388

■ Case 51

Rabushka LS, Kawashima A, Fishman EK. Imaging of the spleen: CT with supplemental MR examination. Radiographics 1994;14(2):307–332

■ Case 52

Boscak A, Shanmuganathan K. Splenic trauma: what is new? Radiol Clin North Am 2012;50(1):105–122

Resteghini N, Nielsen J, Hoimes ML, Karam AR. Delayed splenic rupture presenting 70 days following blunt abdominal trauma. Clin Imaging 2014;38(1):73–74

■ Case 53

Lu M, Weiss C, Fishman EK, Johnson PT, Verde F. Review of visceral aneurysms and pseudoaneurysms. J Comput Assist Tomogr 2015;39(1):1–6

■ Case 54

Dobritz M, Nömayr A, Bautz W, Fellner FA. Gamna-Gandy bodies of the spleen detected with MR imaging: a case report. Magn Reson Imaging 2001;19(9):1249–1251

Vanhoenacker FM, Op de Beeck B, De Schepper AM, Salgado R, Snoeckx A, Parizel PM. Vascular disease of the spleen. Semin Ultrasound CT MR 2007;28(1):35–51

■ Case 55

Feng YM, Huang YC, Tu CW, Kao WS, Tu DG. Distinctive PET/CT features of splenic SANT. Clin Nucl Med 2013;38(12):e465–e466

Pradhan D, Mohanty SK. Sclerosing angiomatoid nodular transformation of the spleen. Arch Pathol Lab Med 2013;137(9):1309–1312

Thipphavong S, Duigenan S, Schindera ST, Gee MS, Philips S. Nonneoplastic, benign, and malignant splenic diseases: cross-sectional imaging findings and rare disease entities. AJR Am J Roentgenol 2014;203(2):315–322

■ Case 56

Thipphavong S, Duigenan S, Schindera ST, Gee MS, Philips S. Nonneoplastic, benign, and malignant splenic diseases: cross-sectional imaging findings and rare disease entities. AJR Am J Roentgenol 2014;203(2):315–322

Willcox TM, Speer RW, Schlinkert RT, Sarr MG. Hemangioma of the spleen: presentation, diagnosis, and management. J Gastrointest Surg 2000;4(6):611–613

■ Case 57

Applegate KE, Goske MJ, Pierce G, Murphy D. Situs revisited: imaging of the heterotaxy syndrome. Radiographics 1999;19(4):837–852, discussion 853–854

Tawfik AM, Batouty NM, Zaky MM, Eladalany MA, Elmokadem AH. Polysplenia syndrome: a review of the relationship with viscero-atrial situs and the spectrum of extra-cardiac anomalies. Surg Radiol Anat 2013;35(8):647–653

■ Case 58

Kim HY, Park JH, Lee YJ, Lee SS, Jeon JJ, Lee KH. Systematic review and meta-analysis of CT features for differentiating complicated and uncomplicated appendicitis. Radiology 2018;287(1):104–115

■ Case 59

Leonards LM, Pahwa A, Patel MK, Petersen J, Nguyen MJ, Jude CM. Neoplasms of the appendix: pictorial review with clinical and pathologic correlation. Radiographics 2017;37(4):1059–1083

■ Case 60

Leonards LM, Pahwa A, Patel MK, Petersen J, Nguyen MJ, Jude CM. Neoplasms of the appendix: pictorial review with clinical and pathologic correlation . Radiographics 2017;37(4):1059–1083

Pickhardt PJ, Levy AD, Rohrmann CA Jr, Kende AI. Primary neoplasms of the appendix: radiologic spectrum of disease with pathologic correlation. Radiographics 2003;23(3):645–662

■ Case 61

Chang S, Choi D, Lee SJ, et al. Neuroendocrine neoplasms of the gastrointestinal tract: classification, pathologic basis, and imaging features. Radiographics 2007;27(6):1667–1679

Frilling A, Akerström G, Falconi M, et al. Neuroendocrine tumor disease: an evolving landscape. Endocr Relat Cancer 2012;19(5):R163–R185

Horton KM, Kamel I, Hofmann L, Fishman EK. Carcinoid tumors of the small bowel: a multitechnique imaging approach. AJR Am J Roentgenol 2004;182(3):559–567

■ Case 62

Ha C, Regan J, Cetindag IB, Ali A, Mellinger JD. Benign esophageal tumors. Surg Clin North Am 2015;95(3):491–514

Zhu X, Zhang XQ, Li BM, Xu P, Zhang KH, Chen J. Esophageal mesenchymal tumors: endoscopy, pathology and immunohistochemistry. World J Gastroenterol 2007;13(5):768–773

■ Case 63

Abdelbaki TN, Abdelsalam WN, ElKayal S. Management modalities in slipped gastric band. Surg Obes Relat Dis 2016;12(3):714–716

Sonavane SK, Menias CO, Kantawala KP, et al. Laparoscopic adjustable gastric banding: what radiologists need to know. Radiographics 2012;32(4):1161–1178

Swenson DW, Pietryga JA, Grand DJ, Chang KJ, Murphy BL, Egglin TK. Gastric band slippage: a case-controlled study comparing new and old radiographic signs of this important surgical complication. AJR Am J Roentgenol 2014;203(1):10–16

■ Case 64

Golabek T, Szymanska A, Szopinski T, et al. Enterovesical fistulae: aetiology, imaging, and management. Gastroenterol Res Pract 2013;2013:617967

Holroyd DJ, Banerjee S, Beavan M, Prentice R, Vijay V, Warren SJ. Colovaginal and colovesical fistulae: the diagnostic paradigm. Tech Coloproctol 2012;16(2):119–126

■ Case 65

Ng KS, Tan AG, Chen KK, Wong SK, Tan HM. CT features of primary epiploic appendagitis. Eur J Radiol 2006;59(2):284–288

Singh AK, Gervais DA, Hahn PF, Sagar P, Mueller PR, Novelline RA. Acute epiploic appendagitis and its mimics. Radiographics 2005;25(6):1521–1534

■ Case 66

Boland GW, Lee MJ, Cats AM, Gaa JA, Saini S, Mueller PR. Antibiotic-induced diarrhea: specificity of abdominal CT for the diagnosis of Clostridium difficile disease. Radiology 1994;191(1):103–106

Kirkpatrick ID, Greenberg HM. Evaluating the CT diagnosis of Clostridium difficile colitis: should CT guide therapy? AJR Am J Roentgenol 2001;176(3):635–639

■ Case 67

Nigri G, Petrucciani N, Giannini G, et al. Giant colonic diverticulum: clinical presentation, diagnosis and treatment: systematic review of 166 cases. World J Gastroenterol 2015;21(1):360–368

Zeina A-R, Mahamid A, Nachtigal A, Ashkenazi I, Shapira-Rootman M. Giant colonic diverticulum: radiographic and MDCT characteristics. Insights Imaging 2015;6(6):659–664

■ Case 68

Cyrany J, Rejchrt S, Kopacova M, Bures J. Buried bumper syndrome: A complication of percutaneous endoscopic gastrostomy. World J Gastroenterol 2016;22(2):618–627

■ Case 69

Chakraborty A, Ayoob A, DiSantis D. Bird's beak sign. Abdom Imaging 2015;40(8):3338–3339

Vandendries C, Jullès MC, Boulay-Coletta I, Loriau J, Zins M. Diagnosis of colonic volvulus: findings on multidetector CT with three-dimensional reconstructions. Br J Radiol 2010;83(995):983–990

■ Case 70

Moore CJ, Corl FM, Fishman EK. CT of cecal volvulus: unraveling the image. AJR Am J Roentgenol 2001;177(1):95–98

Vandendries C, Jullès MC, Boulay-Coletta I, Loriau J, Zins M. Diagnosis of colonic volvulus: findings on multidetector CT with three-dimensional reconstructions. Br J Radiol 2010;83(995):983–990

■ Case 71

Johnson CD, MacCarty RL, Welch TJ, et al. Comparison of the relative sensitivity of CT colonography and double-contrast barium enema for screen detection of colorectal polyps. Clin Gastroenterol Hepatol 2004;2(4):314–321

Pickhardt PJ. Screening CT colonography: how I do it. AJR Am J Roentgenol 2007;189(2):290–298

Pickhardt PJ, Kim DH. CT colonography: pitfalls in interpretation. Radiol Clin North Am 2013;51(1):69–88

■ Case 72

Geffroy Y, Rodallec MH, Boulay-Coletta I, Jullès MC, Ridereau-Zins C, Zins M. Multidetector CT angiography in acute gastrointestinal bleeding: why, when, and how. Radiographics 2011;31(3):E35–E46

Wells ML, Hansel SL, Bruining DH, et al. CT for evaluation of acute gastrointestinal bleeding. Radiographics 2018;38(4):1089–1107

■ Case 73

Gupta P, Debi U, Sinha SK, Prasad KK. Primary versus secondary achalasia: New signs on barium esophagogram. Indian J Radiol Imaging 2015;25(3):288–295

Pandolfino JE, Gawron AJ. Achalasia: a systematic review. JAMA 2015;313(18):1841–1852

■ Case 74

Alexander JA. Endoscopic and radiologic findings in eosinophilic esophagitis. Gastrointest Endosc Clin N Am 2018;28(1):47–57

Diniz LO, Putnum PE, Towbin AJ. Fluoroscopic findings in pediatric eosinophilic esophagitis. Pediatr Radiol 2012;42(6):721–727

■ Case 75

Lazarus DE, Slywotsky C, Bennett GL, Megibow AJ, Macari M. Frequency and relevance of the "small-bowel feces" sign on CT in patients with small-bowel obstruction. AJR Am J Roentgenol 2004;183(5):1361–1366

Paulson EK, Thompson WM. Review of small-bowel obstruction: the diagnosis and when to worry. Radiology 2015;275(2):332–342

■ Case 76

Kozar RA, Crandall M, Shanmuganathan K, et al; AAST Patient Assessment Committee. Organ injury scaling 2018 update: Spleen, liver, and kidney. J Trauma Acute Care Surg 2018;85(6):1119–1122

Yoon W, Jeong YY, Kim JK, et al. CT in blunt liver trauma. Radiographics 2005;25(1):87–104

■ Case 77

Carucci LR, Turner MA. Dysphagia revisited: common and unusual causes. Radiographics 2015;35(1):105–122

Mantsopoulos K, Psychogios G, Karatzanis A, et al. Clinical relevance and prognostic value of radiographic findings in Zenker's diverticulum. Eur Arch Otorhinolaryngol 2014;271(3):583–588

Tao TY, Menias CO, Herman TE, McAlister WH, Balfe DM. Easier to swallow: pictorial review of structural findings of the pharynx at barium pharyngography. Radiographics 2013;33(7):e189–e208

■ Case 78

Gupta S, Levine MS, Rubesin SE, Katzka DA, Laufer I. Usefulness of barium studies for differentiating benign and malignant strictures of the esophagus. AJR Am J Roentgenol 2003;180(3):737–744

Iyer RB, Silverman PM, Tamm EP, Dunnington JS, DuBrow RA. Diagnosis, staging, and follow-up of esophageal cancer. AJR Am J Roentgenol 2003;181(3):785–793

■ Case 79

Gourgiotis S, Vougas V, Germanos S, Baratsis S. Acute gastric volvulus: diagnosis and management over 10 years. Dig Surg 2006;23(3):169–172

Guniganti P, Bradenham CH, Raptis C, Menias CO, Mellnick VM. CT of gastric emergencies. Radiographics 2015;35(7):1909–1921

Rashid F, Thangarajah T, Mulvey D, Larvin M, Iftikhar SY. A review article on gastric volvulus: a challenge to diagnosis and management. Int J Surg 2010;8(1):18–24

■ Case 80

Kang HC, Menias CO, Gaballah AH, et al. Beyond the GIST: mesenchymal tumors of the stomach. Radiographics 2013;33(6):1673–1690

■ Case 81

Ba-Ssalamah A, Prokop M, Uffmann M, Pokieser P, Teleky B, Lechner G. Dedicated multidetector CT of the stomach: spectrum of diseases. Radiographics 2003;23(3):625–644

■ Case 82

Chen CY, Jaw TS, Kuo YT, Hsu JS, Liu GC. Differentiation of gastric ulcers with MDCT. Abdom Imaging 2007;32(6):688–693

Chen CY, Kuo YT, Lee CH, et al. Differentiation between malignant and benign gastric ulcers: CT virtual gastroscopy versus optical gastroendoscopy. Radiology 2009;252(2):410–417

Tonolini M, Ierardi AM, Bracchi E, Magistrelli P, Vella A, Carrafiello G. Non-perforated peptic ulcer disease: multidetector CT findings, complications, and differential diagnosis. Insights Imaging 2017;8(5):455–469

■ Case 83

Mathenge N, Osiro S, Rodriguez II, Salib C, Tubbs RS, Loukas M. Superior mesenteric artery syndrome and its associated gastrointestinal implications. Clin Anat 2014;27(8):1244–1252

Rabie ME, Ogunbiyi O, Al Qahtani AS, Taha SB, El Hadad A, El Hakeem I. Superior mesenteric artery syndrome: clinical and radiological considerations. Surg Res Pract 2015;2015:628705

Sinagra E, Raimondo D, Albano D, et al. Superior mesenteric artery syndrome: clinical, endoscopic, and radiological findings. Gastroenterol Res Pract 2018;2018:1937416

■ Case 84

Lam-Himlin D, Arnold CA, De Petris G. Gastric polyps and polyposis syndromes. Diagn Histopathol 2014;20(1):1–11

Tomas C, Soyer P, Dohan A, Dray X, Boudiaf M, Hoeffel C. Update on imaging of Peutz-Jeghers syndrome. World J Gastroenterol 2014;20(31):10864–10875

■ Case 85

Angthong W, Jiarakoop K, Tangtiang K. Differentiation of benign and malignant ampullary obstruction by multi-row detector CT. Jpn J Radiol 2018;36(8):477–488

Hennedige TP, Neo WT, Venkatesh SK. Imaging of malignancies of the biliary tract- an update. Cancer Imaging 2014;14:14

Nikolaidis P, Hammond NA, Day K, et al. Imaging features of benign and malignant ampullary and periampullary lesions. Radiographics 2014;34(3):624–641

■ Case 86

Heffernan C, Pachter HL, Megibow AJ, Macari M. Stercoral colitis leading to fatal peritonitis: CT findings. AJR Am J Roentgenol 2005;184(4):1189–1193

Ünal E, Onur MR, Balcı S, Görmez A, Akpınar E, Böge M. Stercoral colitis: diagnostic value of CT findings. Diagn Interv Radiol 2017;23(1):5–9

Wu CH, Huang CC, Wang LJ, et al. Value of CT in the discrimination of fatal from non-fatal stercoral colitis. Korean J Radiol 2012;13(3):283–289

■ Case 87

Ghai S, Pattison J, Ghai S, O'Malley ME, Khalili K, Stephens M. Primary gastrointestinal lymphoma: spectrum of imaging findings with pathologic correlation. Radiographics 2007;27(5):1371–1388

Lewis RB, Mehrotra AK, Rodríguez P, Manning MA, Levine MS. From the radiologic pathology archives: gastrointestinal lymphoma: radiologic and pathologic findings. Radiographics 2014;34(7):1934–1953

Lo Re G, Federica V, Midiri F, et al. Radiological features of gastrointestinal lymphoma. Gastroenterol Res Pract 2016;2016:2498143

Sokhandon F, Al-Katib S, Bahoura L, Copelan A, George D, Scola D. Multidetector CT enterography of focal small bowel lesions: a radiological-pathological correlation. Abdom Radiol (NY) 2017;42(5):1319–1341

■ Case 88

Scheirey CD, Scholz FJ, Shortsleeve MJ, Katz DS. Angiotensin-converting enzyme inhibitor-induced small-bowel angioedema: clinical and imaging findings in 20 patients. AJR Am J Roentgenol 2011;197(2):393–398

Sugi MD, Menias CO, Lubner MG, et al. CT Findings of acute small-bowel entities . Radiographics 2018;38(5): 1352–1369

■ **Case 89**

Hepgur M, Ahluwalia MS, Anne N, et al. Medical management of pneumatosis intestinalis in patients undergoing allogeneic blood and marrow transplantation. Bone Marrow Transplant 2011;46(6):876–879

Ho LM, Paulson EK, Thompson WM. Pneumatosis intestinalis in the adult: benign to life-threatening causes. AJR Am J Roentgenol 2007;188(6):1604–1613

St Peter SD, Abbas MA, Kelly KA. The spectrum of pneumatosis intestinalis. Arch Surg 2003;138(1):68–75

■ **Case 90**

Gore RM, Silvers RI, Thakrar KH, et al. Bowel obstruction. Radiol Clin North Am 2015;53(6):1225–1240

Hollerweger A, Rieger S, Mayr N, Mittermair C, Schaffler G. Strangulating closed-loop obstruction: sonographic signs. Ultraschall Med 2016;37(3):271–276

Makar RA, Bashir MR, Haystead CM, et al. Diagnostic performance of MDCT in identifying closed loop small bowel obstruction. Abdom Radiol (NY) 2016;41(7):1253–1260

■ **Case 91**

De Gaetano AM, Lafortune M, Patriquin H, De Franco A, Aubin B, Paradis K. Cavernous transformation of the portal vein: patterns of intrahepatic and splanchnic collateral circulation detected with Doppler sonography. AJR Am J Roentgenol 1995;165(5):1151–1155

Elsayes KM, Shaaban AM, Rothan SM, et al. A comprehensive approach to hepatic vascular disease . Radiographics 2017;37(3):813–836

Kuy S, Dua A, Rieland J, Cronin DC II. Cavernous transformation of the portal vein. J Vasc Surg 2016;63(2):529

■ **Case 92**

Kim YH, Blake MA, Harisinghani MG, et al. Adult intestinal intussusception: CT appearances and identification of a causative lead point. Radiographics 2006;26(3):733–744

■ **Case 93**

Kamaya A, Federle MP, Desser TS. Imaging manifestations of abdominal fat necrosis and its mimics. Radiographics 2011;31(7):2021–2034

Tonerini M, Calcagni F, Lorenzi S, Scalise P, Grigolini A, Bemi P. Omental infarction and its mimics: imaging features of acute abdominal conditions presenting with fat stranding greater than the degree of bowel wall thickening. Emerg Radiol 2015;22(4):431–436

van Breda Vriesman AC, Puylaert JB; van Breda. Epiploic appendagitis and omental infarction: pitfalls and look-alikes. Abdom Imaging 2002;27(1):20–28

■ **Case 94**

Al-Bawardy B, Barlow JM, Vasconcelos RN, et al. Cross-sectional imaging in refractory celiac disease. Abdom Radiol (NY) 2017;42(2):389–395

Scholz FJ, Afnan J, Behr SC. CT findings in adult celiac disease. Radiographics 2011;31(4):977–992

■ **Case 95**

Leung RS, Biswas SV, Duncan M, Rankin S. Imaging features of von Hippel-Lindau disease. Radiographics 2008;28(1):65–79, quiz 323

■ **Case 96**

Baxi AJ, Chintapalli K, Katkar A, Restrepo CS, Betancourt SL, Sunnapwar A. Multimodality imaging findings in carcinoid tumors: a head-to-toe spectrum. Radiographics 2017;37(2):516–536

Bonekamp D, Raman SP, Horton KM, Fishman EK. Role of computed tomography angiography in detection and staging of small bowel carcinoid tumors. World J Radiol 2015;7(9):220–235

■ **Case 97**

Braschi-Amirfarzan M, Keraliya AR, Krajewski KM, et al. Role of imaging in management of desmoid-type fibromatosis: a primer for radiologists. Radiographics 2016;36(3):767–782

Lotfi AM, Dozois RR, Gordon H, et al. Mesenteric fibromatosis complicating familial adenomatous polyposis: predisposing factors and results of treatment. Int J Colorectal Dis 1989;4(1):30–36

■ Case 98

Kim CK, Park BK, Ha H. Gossypiboma in abdomen and pelvis: MRI findings in four patients. AJR Am J Roentgenol 2007;189(4):814–817

Moomjian LN, Clayton RD, Carucci LR. A spectrum of entities that may mimic abdominopelvic abscesses requiring image-guided drainage. Radiographics 2018;38(4):1264–1281

■ Case 99

Cronin CG, O'Connor M, Lohan DG, et al. Imaging of the gastrointestinal complications of systemic chemotherapy. Clin Radiol 2009;64(7):724–733

Rodrigues FG, Dasilva G, Wexner SD. Neutropenic enterocolitis. World J Gastroenterol 2017;23(1):42–47

■ Case 100

Furukawa A, Saotome T, Yamasaki M, et al. Cross-sectional imaging in Crohn disease. Radiographics 2004;24(3):689–702

Index

Locators refer to case number. Locators in boldface indicate primary diagnosis.